Interstitial Lung Diseases

Edited by Jelena Stojšić

Published in London, United Kingdom

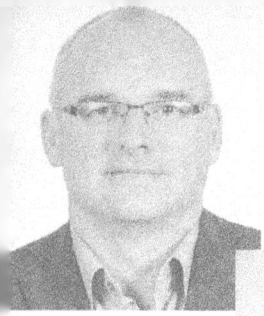
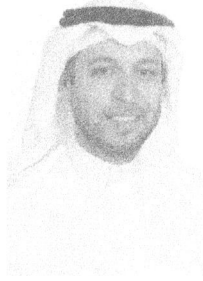
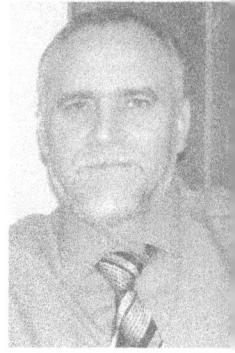
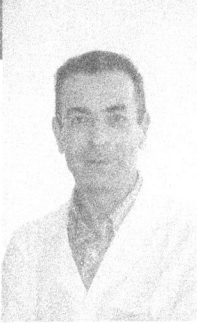
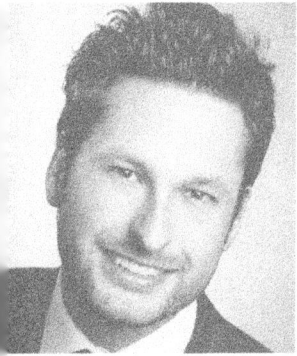
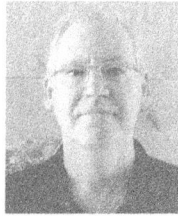
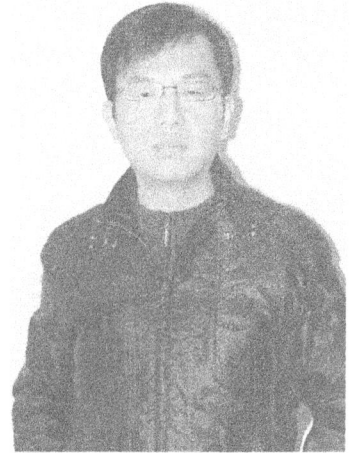

IntechOpen

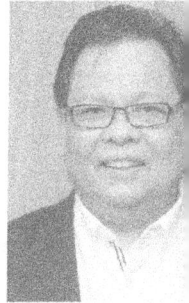
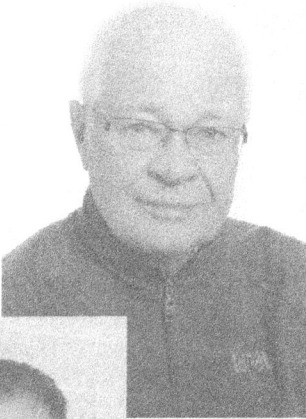
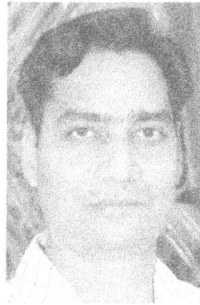
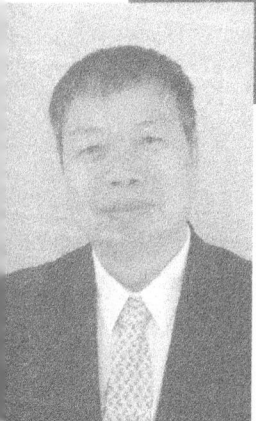
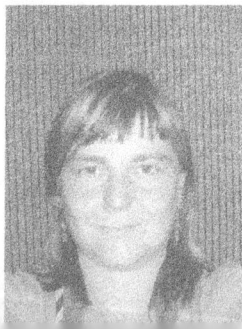
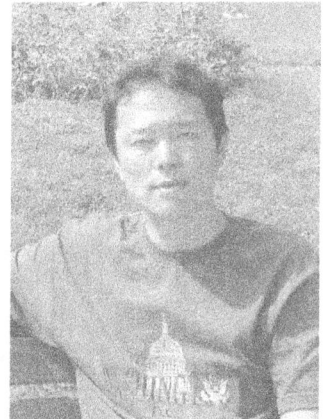

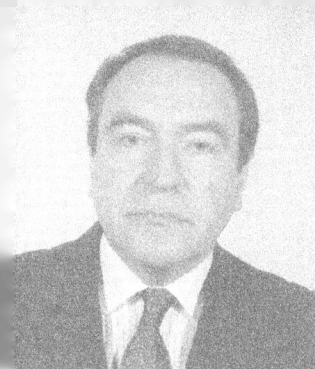

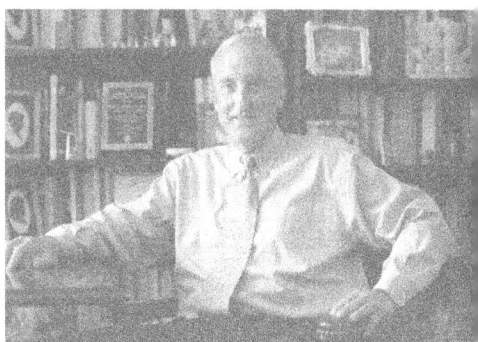

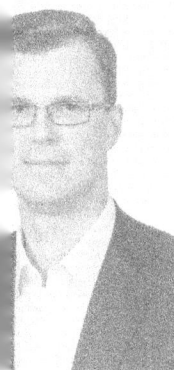

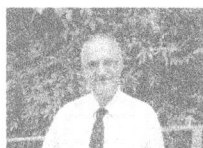

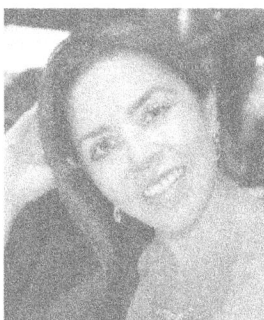

Supporting open minds since 2005

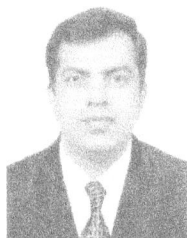

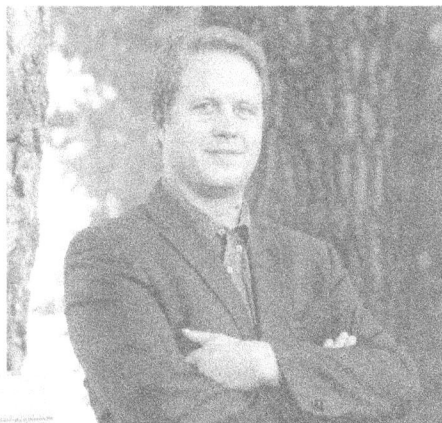

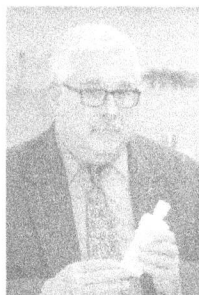

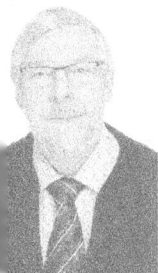

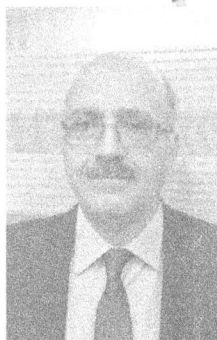

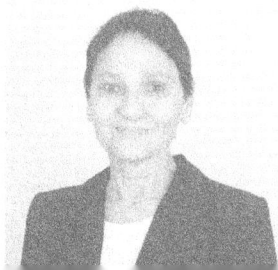

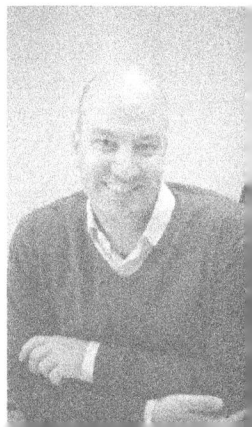

Interstitial Lung Diseases
http://dx.doi.org/10.5772/intechopen.79991
Edited by Jelena Stojšić

Contributors
Munekazu Yamakuchi, Koichi Takagi, Teruto Hashiguchi, Hiromasa Inoue, Kamyar Afshar, Brandon Nokes, Eugene Golts, Sandra Lindstedt, Mohammed Fakhro, Elena Dantes, Emanuela Tudorache, Man Milena Adina, Jelena Stojšić

Notice
Statements and opinions expressed in the chapters are these of the individual contributors and not necessarily those of the editors or publisher. No responsibility is accepted for the accuracy of information contained in the published chapters. The publisher assumes no responsibility for any damage or injury to persons or property arising out of the use of any materials, instructions, methods or ideas contained in the book.

First published in London, United Kingdom, 2019 by IntechOpen
IntechOpen is the global imprint of INTECHOPEN LIMITED, registered in England and Wales, registration number: 11086078, The Shard, 25th floor, 32 London Bridge Street London, SE19SG – United Kingdom
Printed in Croatia

British Library Cataloguing-in-Publication Data
A catalogue record for this book is available from the British Library

Additional hard and PDF copies can be obtained from orders@intechopen.com

Interstitial Lung Diseases
Edited by Jelena Stojšić
p. cm.
Print ISBN 978-1-83881-875-3
Online ISBN 978-1-83881-876-0
eBook (PDF) ISBN 978-1-83881-877-7

We are IntechOpen,
the world's leading publisher of
Open Access books
Built by scientists, for scientists

4,300+

Open access books available

117,000+

International authors and editors

130M+

Downloads

Our authors are among the

151

Countries delivered to

Top 1%

most cited scientists

12.2%

Contributors from top 500 universities

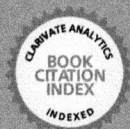

Interested in publishing with us?
Contact book.department@intechopen.com

Numbers displayed above are based on latest data collected.
For more information visit www.intechopen.com

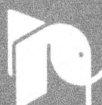

Meet the editor

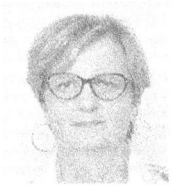

Jelena Stojšić, PhD has been a thoracic pathologist for 25 years. Her major interest is in the field of lung pathology, particularly lung cancer and interstitial lung diseases. She wrote her PhD thesis on reconizing the link between molecular pathways in lung cancer and transport pumps involved in reflux of chemotherapeutics from malignant cells. In daily practice, Dr. Stojšić uses morphology and immunoprofiling to diagnose lung cancer and personalize therapy for her patients.

Contents

Preface

Interstitial lung diseases are rare diffuse lung diseases characterized by specific radiological and pathohistological findings. This book is an attempt to better understand these very specific lung diseases at the molecular level and thus understand and interpret changes in the lung parenchyma and correlate with radiological and pathological findings and therapeutic modalities. This book also includes information on lung transplantation as the most current approach to the treatment of interstitial lung diseases in all stages including the end stage. A special chapter is devoted to the physical therapy of patients with these lung diseases. This book is intended for all doctors who deal with diagnosis and treatment of interstitial lung diseases, as a manual for everyday and practical literature.

I would like to thank all my colleagues who devoted their effort and time in shaping and writing their chapters. I wish them great success in their work.

Jelena Stojšić, MD PhD
Department of Thoracopulmonary Pathology,
Service of Pathology,
Clinical Center of Serbia,
Belgrade, Serbia

Chapter 1

Introductory Chapter: Diagnosis of Interstitial Lung Disease

Jelena Stojšić

1. Introduction

Interstitial lung diseases are rare diffuse lung disease characterized by a specific clinical picture and radiological (imaging) and pathohistological findings. It is considered that these diseases represent about 15% of all respiratory diseases [1].

Diffuse changes of the lung parenchyma in each type of these diseases are characterized by various morphological patterns which are reflected by a different imaging finding and a specific clinical picture [2–4]. The clinical picture at an early stage of the disease is not specific, and it is hard to suspect interstitial lung disease. Symptoms of interstitial lung disease are dry cough, short breath, fever, and fatigue. A specific high resolution - computed tomographyn (HR-CT) finding indicates an interstitial lung disease which is proven by biopsy. Transbronchial biopsy primarily excludes specific granulomatous lung diseases, primary malignancy and metastatic as well as eosinophilic pneumonia, alveolar proteinosis, and pulmonary histiocytosis. If a bioptized lung sample has nonspecific morphological pattern, it is necessary to perform an open lung biopsy or video-assisted thoracoscopic surgery (VATS). Open lung biopsy procedure requires a multidisciplinary approach that includes a chest surgeon. An agreement on taking large number of lung tissue samples characterized by change evolution increases the efficiency and accuracy of the diagnosis [5].

Integrated clinical and radiological data help the pathologist to establish an accurate diagnosis of the type of interstitial lung disease. Besides pulmonologist, radiologist, and pathologist, microbiologist and immunologist also participate in diagnostic procedure [2–4].

2. Pathohistological diagnosis of interstitial lung disease in open lung biopsy

It is necessary to take the entire surgical material for processing and microscopic analysis. Before all, it is necessary to completely instill 10% buffered formalin into the lung parenchyma with a needle for injection but in a moderate amount, in order to not provoke artifacts in the lung parenchyma. In such a manner, alveolar spaces are as if they were in the air-inspiration phase, and also damages on the lung parenchyma caused by a forceps during biopsy performed by a surgeon are avoided. After fixation that lasts 24 h, the entire material is sampled into thin sections which are fixed in the buffered formalin, alcohol, and xylol. After that, they are embedded into paraffin and then cut and stained with a classical hematoxylin-eosin staining.

The pathologist at first performs microscopic examination on a low-powered-field microscope in order to see the distribution of changes, that is, whether they are confluent or not. Then he observes localization of changes and their peribronchial or perivascular presence or connective subpleural, interlobular, or interalveolar septa. On highermicrosopic microscopic field enlargements, the cellularity of changes is noted, as well as the type of cells that contain changes and then the presence and degree of fibrosis. By connective tissue staining, it is desirable to confirm the degree of fibrosis and with other methods to determine type of cells and presence of microorganisms. Immunohistochemical technique can detect the type of cells in the analyzed changes [5].

On the basis of the overall finding, descriptive diagnosis that correlates with the disease entity is made. Diagnosis must correlate with the clinical and imaging picture by the type of change. For this purpose, current classification of interstitial lung diseases is used [5].

The first used classification of interstitial diseases in different subtypes is according to Liebow and Carrington [6]. By consensus of the American Thoracic Society and European Respiratory Society (ATS/ERS), current classification of interstitial lung diseases is determined. This classification defines different clinical-pathological entities according to clinical, radiological, and histological criteria. By using this classification, it is possible to predict the course of the disease, treatment, and outcome. Therapy and monitoring of the disease course require consultative decisions. The medical advisory board consists of experienced pulmonologists, radiologists, and pulmonary pathologists. If the course of the disease is not satisfactory even with applied therapy, treatment may be evaluated, and in exceptional circumstances, archived tissue samples can be reexamined and diagnosis can be changed [1]. In addition to the therapy, in order to improve lung function which is tested by various functional tests, physical therapy is also desirable.

The ATS/ERS classification of these diffuse lung diseases divides them into those of known and those of unknown etiologies [1]. According to ATS/ERS classification, morphological image in the lung parenchyma should correspond to clinical-pathological diagnosis (in this part of the text, insert **Table 1** from the bottom of the text).

Diffuse diseases of known etiology, such as connective tissue diseases or diseases caused by taking some drugs, are less common. Allergic alveolitis or hypersensitivity pneumonitis is a specific entity of generally known etiology. Diseases of unknown etiology, that is, idiopathic diseases such as idiopathic lung disease, non-specific interstitial lung disease, desquamative interstitial pneumonia, respiratory bronchiolitis, organized pneumonia, acute interstitial pneumonia, and lymphoid interstitial pneumonia, are more frequent. This group of diseases includes granulomatosis of which the most common is sarcoidosis characterized by the presence of epithelial, non-necrotizing granulomas [1].

Histological pattern	Clinicopathological diagnosis
Usual interstitial pneumonia (UIP)	Idiopathic pulmonary fibrosis (IPF)/cryptogenic fibrosing alveolitis (CFA)
Nonspecific interstitial pneumonia (NSIP)	Nonspecific pneumonia
Organizing pneumonia	Cryptogenic organizing pneumonia
Diffuse alveolar damage (DAD)	Acute interstitial pneumonia
Desquamative interstitial pneumonia (DIP)	Desquamative interstitial pneumonia
Respiratory bronchiolitis	Respiratory bronchiolitis-interstitial lung disease (RB-ILD)
Lymphocytic interstitial pneumonia (LIP)	Lymphocytic interstitial pneumonia

Table 1.
Morphological image which corresponds to a certain clinical-pathological diagnosis according to the ATS/ERS classification [1].

By using the said formulations, uniformity of the findings is achieved and therapy is specified. If good treatment results fail, it comes to a stage known as "end-stage lung disease." In such a case, lung transplantation is proposed which lately requires a special chapter in each textbook about these diseases. Selection of the transplantation type (single, bilateral, or heart-lungs) depends on the type of interstitial lung disease and other factors. The success of transplantation depends on the type of organism reaction on the presence of the transplanted lung or the type of rejection which can be subacute, acute, and chronic. Changes in rejection reactions are localized around the blood vessels of the lungs or bronchi. The intensity of rejection reaction depends on the extent of the changes spreading in the pulmonary interstitium and the type of inflammatory infiltrate. Prevention and treatment of rejection are regulated by immunosuppressive drugs. Therefore, it is necessary to control the presence of microorganisms in the transplanted lung by microbiological tests and transbronchial biopsy [7–9].

However, the future of the treatment of interstitial lung diseases depends on the molecular changes in the cells found in the lesions. miRNAs profiling in lung tissue in various interstitial lung diseases in a variety of cells that contain lung lesions: endothelium, alveolar epithelium, inflammatory cells, fibroblast and myofibroblast. This profiling can determine the type of therapy and their outcome or success.

Author details

Jelena Stojšić
Department of Thoracopulmonary Pathology, Service of Pathology, Clinical Center of Serbia, Belgrade, Serbia

*Address all correspondence to: dr.jelenastoj@gmail.com

IntechOpen

References

[1] American Thoracic Society/European Respiratory Society International Multidisciplinary Consensus Classification of the idiopathic inetrstitial pneumonias. American Journal of Respiratory and Critical Care Medicine. 2002;**165**:277-304

[2] Cottin V. Interstitial lung disease. European Respiratory Review. 2013;**22**:26-32

[3] Flaherty KR, King TE Jr, Raghu G, Lynch JP 3rd, Colby TV, Travis WD, et al. Idiopathic interstitial pneumonia: What is the effect of a multidisciplinary approach to diagnosis? American Journal of Respiratory and Critical Care Medicine. 2004;**170**:904-910

[4] Thomeer M, Demedts M, Behr J, Buhl R, Costabel U, Flower CD, et al. Multidisciplinary observer agreement in the diagnosis and of idiopathic pulmonary fibrosis. The European Respiratory Journal. 2008;**31**:585-591

[5] Leslie KO. Pathology of interstitial lung disease. Clinics in Chest Medicine. 2004;**25**:657-703

[6] Liebow AA, Carringotn CB. In: Simon M, Potchen EJ, Lemay M, editors. The Interstitial Pneumonias, Frontiers of Pulmonary Radiology. New York: Grune and Strattin; 1969. pp. 102-141

[7] Roden AC, Aisner DL, Allen TC, Aubry MC, Barrios RJ, Beasley MB, et al. Diagnosis of acute cellular rejection and antibody-mediated rejection on lung transplant biopsies: A perspective from members of the pulmonary pathology society. Archives of Pathology & Laboratory Medicine. 2017;**141**(3):437-444

[8] Roden AC, Maleszewski JJ, Yi ES, Jenkins SM, Gandhi MJ, Scott JP, et al. Reproducibility of complement 4d deposition by immunofluorescence and immunohistochemistry in lung allograft biopsies. The Journal of Heart and Lung Transplantation. 2014;**33**(12):1223-1232

[9] Calabrese F, Alessandrini L, Loy M, Marulli G, Balestro E, Perissinotto E, et al. Comparison between referral diagnosis of patients requiring transplantation and pathologic diagnosis of native lungs. The Journal of Heart and Lung Transplantation. 2009;**28**(11):1135-1140

Chapter 2

The Role of miRNAs in Idiopathic Pulmonary Fibrosis

Koichi Takagi, Munekazu Yamakuchi, Teruto Hashiguchi and Hiromasa Inoue

Abstract

Idiopathic pulmonary fibrosis (IPF) is a genetic heterogeneous disease with high mortality and poor prognosis. IPF is characterized by persistent fibroblasts and relentless accumulation of collagen matrix. Epithelial-mesenchymal transition (EMT) and endothelial-to-mesenchymal transition (EndoMT) contribute to the progression of the fibrotic process. There are some therapeutic drugs that delay this progress, but eradicative medicine does not exist yet. MicroRNAs (miRNAs) are short single-stranded RNAs that regulate posttranscriptional silencing. Recent reports have shown that miRNAs play important roles in the development of IPF, as different expression levels of miRNAs in blood and lung tissue from IPF patients were closely associated with the occurrence of IPF disease. In this chapter, we will discuss the role of miRNAs in the pathogenesis, diagnosis, and treatment of IPF. In particular, we will focus on the regulation of EMT/EndoMT by miRNAs.

Keywords: IPF, miRNA, EndoMT, EMT

1. Introduction

1.1 Overview of idiopathic pulmonary fibrosis

Idiopathic pulmonary fibrosis (IPF) is a genetic heterogeneous disease with high mortality and poor prognosis that is characterized by progressive scarring of the pulmonary parenchyma, which leads to progressive loss of lung function with dyspnea and hypoxemia, and ultimately respiratory failure and death. IPF is a specific form of chronic, progressive, fibrosing interstitial pneumonia of unknown cause. Disease pathogenesis involves airway tissue remodeling through the excess deposition of extracellular matrix (ECM) proteins and the formation of fibroblastic foci, evident by histology [1]. These events are occurred mainly by continuous damage to the lung epithelium, which destroys the basement membrane and activates myofibroblasts. Myofibroblasts may not only come from resident or circulating fibroblasts but also be brought by epithelial cells transdifferentiated through epithelial-mesenchymal transition (EMT) [2]. Signaling through the TGF-β pathway is thought to underlie many of these changes [3].

According to the 2018 joint statement by the American Thoracic Society (ATS), European Respiratory Society (ERS), Latin America Thoracic Association (ALAT), and Japanese Respiratory Society (JRS) [4], the diagnosis of IPF can be secured by exclusion of other known causes of interstitial lung disease (ILD) and either the presence of high resolution computed tomography (HRCT) pattern of usual inter-stitial pneumonia (UIP) or specific combinations of HRCT patterns and histopa-thology patterns in patients subjected to lung tissue sampling. Any plausible cause of secondary interstitial involvement should be excluded by a thorough medical his-tory and other procedures such as laboratory tests or bronchoalveolar lavage (BAL) when necessary. If a specific diagnosis is not made or no potential cause for ILD is identified, then clinical findings and HRCT are considered during multidisciplinary discussion among different experts (including clinicians, radiologists, pathologists, rheumatologists, and thoracic surgeons in selected cases) [4].

1.2 Overview of miRNAs

MicroRNAs (miRNAs) are short single-stranded RNA molecules of 19–25 nucleotides in length that mediate posttranscriptional gene silencing of target genes [5]. MiRNAs have been recognized as a distinct class of small regulatory RNAs in multiple species that regulate a wide variety of functions such as cell proliferation, differentiation, apoptosis, stress response, and immune response [6–8]. MiRNAs regulate the onset and progress of a variety of diseases, such as cancer, infections, and atherosclerosis [9–11]. In lung diseases, many miRNAs contribute to the patho-genesis. For instance, miR-424/503 regulates the progression of pulmonary hyper-tension (PH) [12, 13]. miR-424/503 expression is reduced in the pulmonary artery of PH patients [13]. One of the targets of miR-424/503 is *Rictor*, and inhibition of miR-424/503 expression increased the expression of *Rictor*, leading to endothelial-to-mesenchymal transition (EndoMT) and migration of pulmonary artery endo-thelial cells [12]. In allergic asthma, miR-21, miR-126, and miR-145 are upregulated in multiple experimental asthma models [14–16], and miR-221 and miR-485-3p are upregulated in the peripheral blood of pediatric patients with asthma, compared with controls [17].

2. IPF and miRNAs

Profiling of miRNAs in the lung tissue from IPF patients was performed by different groups [18–22]. In IPF lungs, the expression of miR-21 and miR-155 was increased, whereas the expression of let-7a, miR-29, miR-30, and miR-101 was decreased [23–25]. MiR-21 expression was increased in the serum of IPF patients, and its levels correlated with a decrease in lung function [26]. In the miRNA expres-sion profiling of sputum-derived exosomes from IPF patients, 21 miRNAs were dif-ferentially expressed, among which seven (e.g., miR-142-3p and miR-33a-5p) were upregulated and 14 (e.g., Let-7d-5p) were downregulated [27]. In bronchoalveolar lavage fluid (BALF), miR-29a and miR-185 are downregulated in IPF patients [28, 29]. However, little is known about miRNA functions in IPF; much of the functional data has been inferred from chemically induced mouse IPF models. In the lungs of mouse IPF models, miR-21, miR-9, and miR-155 were increased [19, 21, 30], and miR-26, miR-101, miR-139, miR-200, miR-326, miR-489, miR-503, and miR-708 were decreased [24, 31–37]. Furthermore, miR-21 expression was increased in myofibroblasts from IPF lungs, and its inhibition in mouse IPF models attenuated the disease severity [19]. The expression of miR-200 family members was reduced in mouse IPF models and restoration of miR-200c inhibited fibrosis [33]. Similarly, miR-26a was decreased in mouse IPF models and its inhibition caused pulmonary fibrosis, while overexpression repressed fibrotic disease [38]. Finally, miR-326 was decreased in mouse IPF models, and its administration mimicked inhibited TGF-β expression and attenuated fibrosis [34].

3. The role of miRNAs in IPF-contributing cells

Epithelial cells communicate each other via adhesion molecules under physiological condition. Among many adhesion molecules, E-cadherin plays an important role in maintaining tight junctions of epithelial cells. Recurrent and nonresolving injury to lung epithelial cells appears to be a key driver of pulmonary fibrosis. Recent studies have supported the concept that altered alveolar epithelial cell phenotypes, including those produced by increased endoplasmic reticulum stress, predispose to further epithelial cell injury and abnormal repair, facilitating the development of pulmonary fibrosis [39, 40], and thus suggested that the epithelial abnormalities/dysfunction underlying fibrosis should be referred to as reprogramming. The ability of epithelial cells to change into mesenchymal cells through EMT plays an important role in the development of IPF.

Myofibroblasts and related mesenchymal cells are generally accepted as the cells predominantly responsible for fibrotic destruction/distortion of the lung in IPF [41]. Proliferation of fibroblasts and their differentiation into myofibroblasts are important in the development of IPF. The stage of mesenchymal cell differentiation at which IPF myofibroblasts acquire hallmark pathological properties, the mechanisms underlying their pathological differentiation, and the roles of signals from epithelial cells, immune cells, and the matrix in this process has not been fully elucidated and requires further research.

The lung extracellular matrix (ECM) is comprised of collagens, elastin, glycoproteins, and proteoglycans, which serve as structural scaffolding for cells and provide the mechanical stability and elastic recoil necessary for proper lung function. In normal wound healing, myofibroblasts that produce ECM proteins are recruited during the active phase of repair, but are quickly removed via apoptosis once the repair process is underway. Most of the scar matrix subsequently resolves and is replaced by a more permanent tissue. In IPF, myofibroblasts are relatively resistant to apoptosis, and their persistence leads to excessive scarring [42]. A hallmark of IPF is the accumulation of myofibroblasts in clusters called fibroblastic foci and extensive ECM deposition within the interstitium, resulting in destruction of alveolar architecture.

Vascular muscularization driven by repeated small injury is the main pathogenesis of PH, leading to the sustained fibrotic process of intima [43]. Different cellular processes have been described during pulmonary artery remodeling of PH-associated IPF, including endothelial dysfunction [44], EndoMT as a source of myofibroblasts [45], and pulmonary artery smooth muscle proliferation [46].

Monocytes and macrophages have a key role in regulating tissue repair and fibrosis, and several molecular pathways regulating their activity are being investigated as potential treatments for IPF. Macrophages possess many functions that would be expected to promote fibrosis, including fibroblast proliferation [47], regulation of ECM components [48], and secretion of profibrotic cytokines and growth factors. However, macrophages may also possess antifibrotic properties [47, 49]. Several studies have attributed these opposing functions to different macrophage populations distinguished along the lines of classical (M1) and alternative (M2) macrophage activation [50–52], with M1 macrophages being antifibrotic and M2 macrophages being either profibrotic or regulatory.

Adaptive immune responses are involved in the pathological process in IPF patients. Infiltration of activated CD4+ T-cells into IPF lung is often observed before symptoms are developed [53]. Mature dendritic cells also infiltrate in the pulmonary parenchyma of IPF patients [54]. FoxP3 positive regulatory T-cells are diminished in both the circulation and BALF of IPF patients [55].

3.1 Alveolar epithelial cells

miRNA microarray analysis of lung tissue from healthy controls and IPF patients showed that the expression of several let-7 family members was lower in IPF patients [18]. The human let-7 family includes 12 members (let-7-a1, a2, a3, b, c, d, e, f1, f2, g, 1, and miR-98), located on eight different homologous chromosomes [56]. *In vitro* inhibition of let-7d induced an increase in mesenchymal markers in lung epithelial cell lines. The High Mobility Group A2 (*HMGA2*) 3′ UTR has seven conserved sites complementary to the let-7 miRNA [57], and HMGA2 was significantly overexpressed in IPF lungs compared with controls [58]. In lung epithelial cell lines, let-7d regulated *HMGA2* expression, and the increase in *HMGA2* after TGF-β stimulation depended on inhibition of let-7 [18]. HMGA2 facilitates the transcription of *SNAI1* and *TWIST*, the transcriptional repressors of adherens, which are tight and desmosomal junction components, leading to reduced intracellular adhesion. Moreover, it is a mediator of TGF-β-induced EMT. Downregulation of let-7d also led to upregulation of other fibrosis-relevant targets, such as RAS, insulin-like growth factor-1 (IGF-1), and IGF-1 receptor, and thus to the profound and sustained changes in cellular phenotype that are indeed observed in IPF [18] (**Figure 1**).

The expression of miR-26a was significantly decreased in the lungs of mice following the administration of bleomycin [59]. Alignment of miR-26a with the *HMGA2* 3′UTR sequence revealed one potential conserved seed site. Transient introduction of miR-26a into A549 cells, a pulmonary epithelial cell line, led to a significant decrease in HMGA2. However, the reduction in miR-26a expression induced an obvious EMT phenotype in A549 cells together with a clear alteration in certain related proteins, including E-cadherin, vimentin, and α-SMA [59]. Loss of function of miR-26a facilitated lung epithelial cells to transform into myofibroblasts and induce pulmonary fibrosis in mice. Lin28D is also one of the conserved putative target genes of miR-26a. Inhibition of miR-26a induced Lin28D expression and caused an obvious EMT phenotype in A549 cells [31].

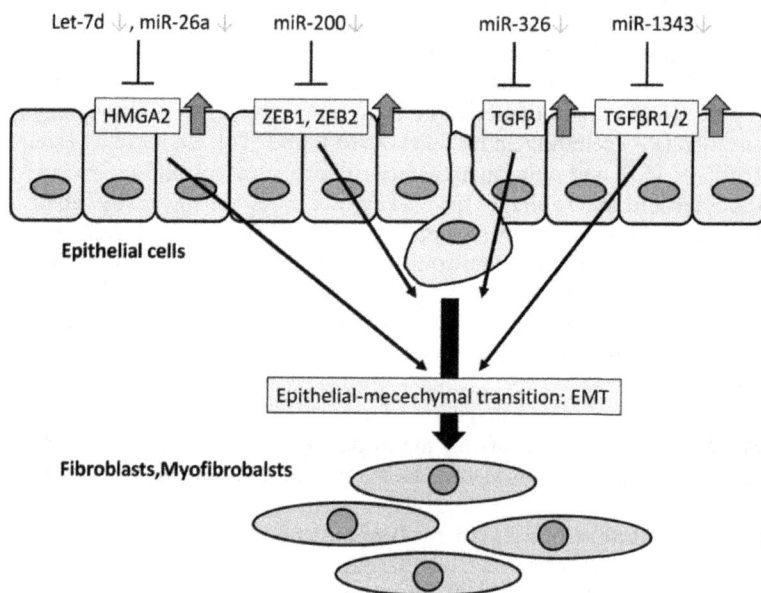

Figure 1.
The role of miRNAs in alveolar epithelial cells for IPF.

The miR-200 family has been suggested to regulate the progression of pulmonary fibrosis by suppressing the EMT of alveolar epithelial cells (AECs). MiR-200 family members correlated with E-cadherin expression in epithelial cells [60, 61] and negatively correlated with ZEB family expression, which has been implicated in EMT [62]. Furthermore, the miR-200 family members have been identified as EMT suppressors through direct targeting of ZEB1 and ZEB2 [63]. MiR-200 is downregulated in the lungs of IPF patients and mouse IPF models [33]. In AECs, overexpression of miR-200, particularly miR-200b and miR-200c, attenuated TGF-β1-induced mesenchymal cell morphological characteristics and TGF-β1-repressed E-cadherin expression [33].

In fibrotic lungs, TGF-β1 is overexpressed in a broad range of cells, including epithelial cells, leading to the dysregulation of normal lung homeostasis by increasing the synthesis and altering the balance of matrix metalloproteinases and their inhibitors [64]. MiR-326 targets the *TGF-β1* 3′UTR, and miR-326 levels inversely correlate with TGF-β1 protein levels in multiple human cell lines and in the lungs of mouse IPF models [34]. Restoration of miR-326 levels by intranasal delivery of miR-326 mimics was sufficient to inhibit TGF-β1 expression and attenuate the fibrotic response in the lungs of mouse IPF models [34]. Furthermore, miR-1343 targets the 3′UTRs of *TGFBR1* and *TGFBR2* and attenuates EMT and fibrogenesis by inhibiting the TGF-β1 pathway in alveolar epithelial cell lines [65].

3.2 Fibroblasts and myofibroblasts

Several studies have shown that some miRNAs including miR-21, miR-29, miR-101, miR-153, miR-154, miR-155, and miR-210 regulate the function of fibroblasts in the lungs (**Figure 2**).

The expression of miR-21 is increased in the lungs of mouse IPF models and of patients with IPF [19]. In mouse IPF models, miR-21 inhibition by lentiviruses encoding anti-miR-21 suppressed morphological markers of pulmonary fibrosis compared with controls [23]. TGF-β1 is the most important profibrogenic cytokine, which increases the expression of miR-21 through SMAD2/3/4 in lung fibroblasts [19] [66]. MiR-21 inhibition inversely regulates TGF-β1-induced ECM protein expression in human pulmonary fibroblast cell lines [23]. Smad7, which inhibits the proliferation of interstitial fibroblasts, is a direct target of miR-21 and negatively correlates with miR-21 in pulmonary fibroblasts [19].

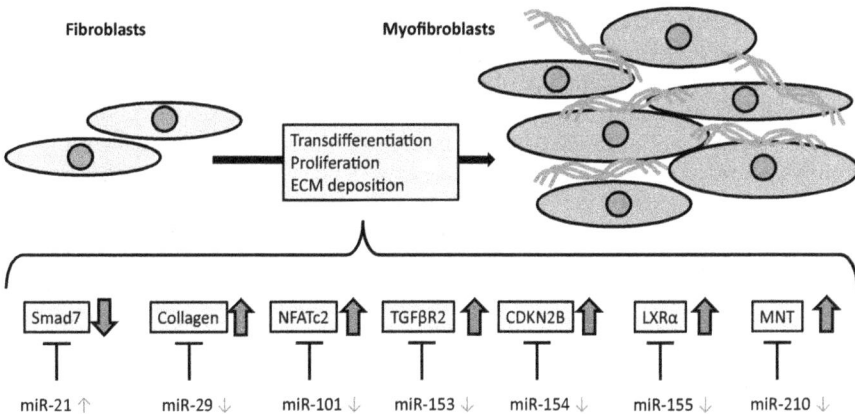

Figure 2.
The role of miRNAs in fibroblasts for IPF.

Members of the miR-29 family, which consists of three mature members, miR-29a, miR-29b, and miR-29c, are among the most downregulated miRNAs in IPF lungs [66]. The expression of miR-29c is also decreased in the lungs of mouse IPF models [67]. MiR-29 has many target genes involved in the composition and regulation of ECM, thus downregulation of miR-29 is capable of contributing to excessive ECM deposition [20, 68]. In human fetal lung fibroblasts, miR-29 suppression upregulated a series of genes, such as TGF-β1 regulated genes and adhesion molecules associated with the fibrotic phenotype [18].

MiR-101 is also one of the most downregulated miRNAs in fibrotic lungs from IPF patients and mouse IPF models [24]. Hypoxia-inducible factors (HIFs) contribute to the pathogenesis of pulmonary fibrosis through Nuclear Factor-Activated T-cell (NFAT) c2 [69]. MiR-101 suppressed WNT5a-induced proliferation of lung fibroblasts via inhibition of NFATc2 signaling by targeting Frizzled receptor 4/6 and attenuated bleomycin-induced pulmonary fibrosis in mouse IPF models [24].

MiR-153 is an intragenic miRNA that is embedded in genes encoding islet-associated protein (IA)-2 and 2β. It has been shown to participate in the pathogenesis of neurodegenerative diseases [70] and inhibit the proliferation and invasion of many types of malignant cells [71]. Furthermore, TGF-β1 downregulates miR-153 expression in lung fibrosis, and miR-153 was downregulated in the fibrotic phase, which was characterized by excessive proliferation of fibroblasts and deposition of ECM in mouse IPF models [72]. However, miR-153 reduced the contractile and migratory activities of fibroblasts. TGFBR2, a transmembrane serine/threonine kinase receptor for TGF-β, has been identified as a direct target of miR-153; moreover, miR-375 regulates SMAD2/3 phosphorylation and the fibrogenic activity of lung fibroblasts through TGFBR2 inhibition [72].

The majority of increased miRNAs in IPF localizes to chromosome 14q32 and is enriched with members of the miR-154 family. TGF-β1 regulates the expression of miRNAs in the 14q32 cluster and induces the expression changes similar to those seen in IPF. TGF-β1 induces cell proliferation through CDK4 and CDKN2B, a CDK4 inhibitor, which is a miR-154 target. Furthermore, TGF-β1-induced increases in proliferation were significantly reduced in the presence of miR-154 inhibitor in fibroblasts, and miR-154-induced changes in proliferation were mediated through the activation of the WNT/β-catenin pathway in fibroblasts [73].

MiR-155 is required for normal immune function [74]. Its overexpression is associated with inflammation, autoimmunity, and cancer [75], whereas miR-155-deficient mice develop age-related airway fibrosis [76]. Liver X receptor alpha (LXRα), which is an oxysterol-activated transcription factor, has a conserved 3′UTR seed-region sequence complementary to miR-155, and inhibition of LXRα ameliorated lung fibrosis in miR-155-deficient mice [77]. However, enforced expression of miR-155 reduced the profibrotic phenotype of IPF and miR-155-deficient fibroblasts [77]. Thus, miR-155 attenuates lung fibrosis through inhibition of LXRα in lung fibroblasts.

The expression of miR-210 has been found to be increased in patients with rapidly progressive IPF, who typically have experienced hypoxia [22]. Consistently, miR-210 was upregulated in IPF fibroblasts in response to hypoxia, and its knockdown suppressed the hypoxia-induced proliferation of IPF fibroblasts. Furthermore, HIF-2α regulated miR-210 expression and miR-210-mediated proliferation of IPF fibroblasts in response to hypoxia. Finally, miR-210 promoted IPF fibroblast proliferation through repression of its downstream target, MNT [78].

3.3 Endothelial cells

PH is frequently seen in IPF patients and is commonly attributed to hypoxic vasoconstriction and capillary destruction. Pathology findings include endothelial proliferation and medial hypertrophy that exceed those expected in the setting of hypoxia [79] (**Figure 3**). HIF-1 activates the transcription of genes encoding angiogenic growth factors, including vascular endothelial growth factor (VEGF), angiopoietin (ANGPT), placental growth factor (PGF), and platelet-derived growth factor (PDGF), which are secreted by hypoxic cells and stimulate endothelial cells, leading to angiogenesis. Furthermore, HIF-1 mediates hypoxia-induced phenotypic changes typical of EndoMT in endothelial cells [80].

ANGPT1 is a ligand for receptor tyrosine kinase Tie2 [81], which is expressed in endothelial cells [82]. ANGPT1-Tie2 signaling has been shown to be involved mainly in angiogenic activity and promoting maturation of blood vessels, and it is regulated by Akt and MAPK signaling [83, 84]. The activation of ANGPT1-Tie2 signaling correlates with the severity of PH [85]. Mir-34a is downregulated in rat pulmonary arterial hypertension models [86], and ANGPT1 and Tie2 are potential targets of miR-34a, as they have a conserved miR-34a seed sequence in their 3′UTR [87]. Overexpression of miR-34a also downregulated the expression of PDGFRA, one of therapeutic targets of IPF, in pulmonary artery smooth muscle cells [86].

EndoMT has been proposed to be another potential source of myofibroblasts. In EndoMT, endothelial cells lose their own markers and obtain mesenchymal phenotype. Silencing of miR-155 directly increased RhoA expression and activity in endothelial cells and affected phosphorylation of the downstream LMK. A selective Rho kinase inhibitor partly suppressed EndoMT, strengthening the notion that RhoA plays a central role in EndoMT. Overexpression of miR-155 suppressed EndoMT, hence miR-155 functions as a negative regulator of RhoA signaling in TGF-β-induced EndoMT [88]. EndoMT has been considered as a source of myofibroblasts in PH [45], and miR-155 is downregulated in IPF lungs. Thus, miR-155 has been suggested to affect PH-associated IPF through inducing EndoMT.

3.4 Inflammatory cells

Macrophages possess many functions that would be expected to promote fibrosis, including regulation of fibroblast proliferation, recruitment, and activation, direct regulation of ECM components, and secretion of profibrotic cytokines and growth factors. There are two opposite characteristic types of functional macrophages; pro-inflammatory (M1) macrophages induced by toll-like receptor (TLR) and T helper type 1 (Th1) signals and anti-inflammatory (M2) macrophages

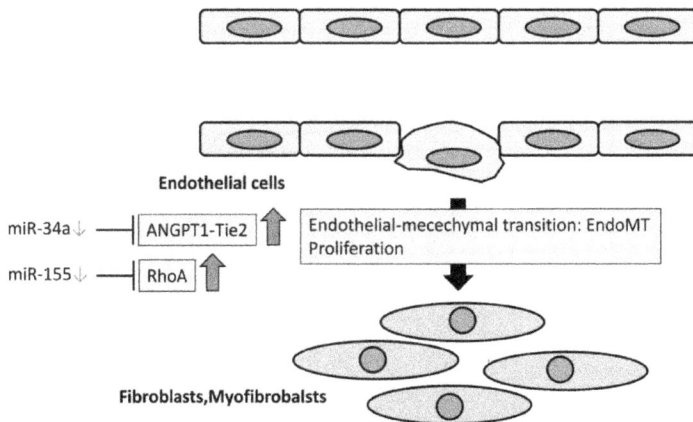

Endothelial cells

miR-34a↓ — ANGPT1-Tie2 ⇧   Endothelial-mecechymal transition: EndoMT
miR-155↓ — RhoA ⇧   Proliferation

Fibroblasts,Myofibrobalsts

Figure 3.
The role of miRNAs in pulmonary endothelial cells for IPF.

activated by Th2 signals [89] [90]. Th2 cytokines, IL-4 and IL-13 (IL-4/IL-13), contribute to extensive tissue fibrosis in mouse models [91], and IL-4/IL-13-induced macrophages activate fibroblasts by secreting pro-fibrogenic cytokines. IL-4/IL-13 induced CCL18 in lung macrophages of IPF patients, and secreted CCL18 increased the production of collagen from fibroblasts [92]. Many transcriptional factors, such as STAT (signal transducers and activator of transcription) family, regulate macrophage polarization. M1 macrophage polarization is controlled via STAT1, and M2 macrophages activation is mediated by STAT6 [93]. To maintain STAT6 phosphorylation, M2 macrophages overcome strong expression of suppressor of cytokine signaling 1 (SOCS1), resulting in the prolongation of fibrogenesis (**Figure 4**).

IL-4/IL-13 induced miR-142-5p expression and suppressed miR-130a-3p expression in macrophages [94]. Transfection of macrophages with either miR-142-5p anti-sense oligonucleotides or miR-130-3p mimics significantly reduced the expression of M2 markers induced by IL-4 and regulated macrophage pro-fibrogenesis [94]. SOCS1 3′UTR has seven conserved sites complementary to miR-142-5p RNA, and PPARγ 3′UTR has seven conserved sites complementary to miR-130a-3p RNA. The expression of SOCS1 is reduced in IPF lungs, and bleomycin-induced lung fibrosis and inflammation were enhanced in SOCS1-deficient mice compared with WT mice [95]. Thus, miR-142-5p and miR-130a-3p regulate pulmonary fibrosis through SOCS1 and PPARγ in macrophages.

Downregulation of miR-185 has been demonstrated in IPF lung tissue and alveolar macrophages [29, 96]. MiR-185 inhibited cell growth and proliferation by directly targeting AKT1 [97]. Downregulation of miR-185 resulted in AKT activation via increased DNMT1 expression, leading to promoter hypermethylation and silencing of *PTEN* [77]. Moreover, miR-185 directly bound and degraded the 3′UTR of *AKT1* mRNA [98]. Finally, TGF-β1 inhibited the expression of miR-185 in macrophages, and thus TGF-β1 signaling has been suggested to induce proliferation and activation of macrophages through inhibition of miR-185 expression [98].

Some lymphocytic cytokines are considered profibrotic with direct effects on fibroblast and myofibroblast activity in IPF. Th1, Th2, and Th17 have been linked to IPF pathogenesis. The Th1 subset produces IL-1α, TNF-α, PDGF, and TGF-β1. The Th2 subset typical interleukins are IL-4 and IL-13, which are directly involved in fibroblast activation and ECM production. The Th17 subset indirectly promotes fibrosis by increasing TGF-β1 levels, and it is positively regulated by TGF-β1,

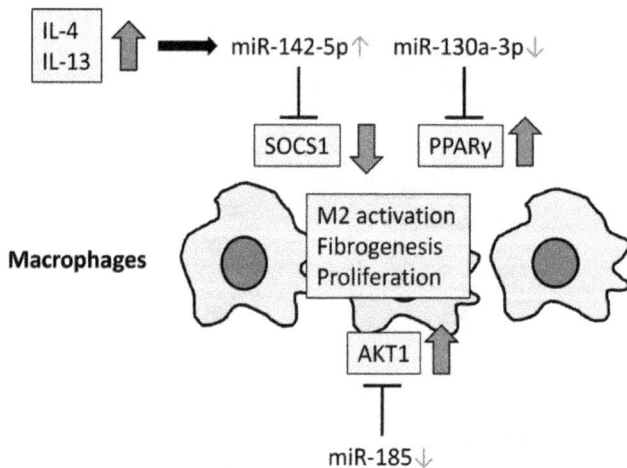

Figure 4.
The role of miRNAs in macrophages for IPF.

creating a positive feedback loop [99]. In both BALF and the peripheral blood of IPF patients, the number of CD4 + CD25 + FOXP3+ regulatory T-cells (Tregs) is decreased compared with healthy people. Thus, Tregs' numerical and functional deficiency may play a central role in the initial phases of IPF pathogenesis [55].

In CD4+ T cells, the level of miR-155 expression is positively associated with the expression of the Th2 cytokines, IL-5 and IL-13, and miR-155 suppresses inhibitors of cytokine production including SOCS1 [100]. However, Foxp3 inhibition significantly decreased miR-146a expression in Tregs. The target gene of miR-146a is TNF receptor-associated factor 6 (TRAF6). Foxp3 and miR-146a have been suggested to regulate colonic inflammation and fibrosis by negatively regulating TRAF6 [101].

4. Conclusions

IPF is a heterogeneous disease that is affected and developed by various genetic backgrounds and environments. The recent development and approval of antifibrotic agents such as nintedanib and pirfenidone, both of which reduced the lung function decline rate in IPF patients in clinical trials, offer hope that it may be possible to alter the increased mortality associated with IPF; however, these therapeutic effects are not sufficient for curing the disease. To reveal new therapeutic IPF targets, genetic screening of IPF patients, including miRNAs, is an effective option. Over the past decade, the role of miRNAs in both promoting and alleviating chronic respiratory disease has become increasingly apparent. In IPF, some miRNAs have been indicated to be associated with EMT, EndoMT, fibrocyte differentiation, or ECM deposition. Investigation of miRNAs and their target genes associated with IPF may lead to new therapy. However, there have been some problems with applying miRNAs in the clinical scene: (1) multiple groups performing studies with similar experimental conditions have reported different and often contrasting results. Hence, collection methods and specimen parts need to be standardized, and better assays are needed for high-confidence miRNA measurements. (2) It is not clear whether miRNA misregulation is a direct cause of disease or an indirect result of gene regulatory processes. Most studies did not attempt to establish the necessity and sufficiency of the miRNA under investigation. (3) It is still difficult to interfere with miRNA expression in the human body, and it is possible that such interference will cause unexpected adverse reactions. (4) It has not been established how to introduce miRNAs into target cells safely and effectively, and the cost of this treatment will probably be high. Thus, miRNAs are still insufficient to be used as therapeutic targets in the clinical scene. Nevertheless, miRNAs may be important tools as IPF biomarkers. To use miRNAs clinically, further studies are necessary to elucidate the association between miRNAs and IPF.

Author details

Koichi Takagi[1], Munekazu Yamakuchi[2*], Teruto Hashiguchi[2] and Hiromasa Inoue[2]

1 Department of Pulmonary Medicine, Kagoshima University Graduate School of Medical and Dental Sciences, Kagoshima, Japan

2 Department of Laboratory and Vascular Medicine, Kagoshima University Graduate School of Medical and Dental Sciences, Kagoshima, Japan

*Address all correspondence to: munekazu@m.kufm.kagoshima-u.ac.jp

IntechOpen

References

[1] Fernandez IE, Eickelberg O. New cellular and molecular mechanisms of lung injury and fibrosis in idiopathic pulmonary fibrosis. Lancet. 2012;**380**(9842):680-688. DOI: 10.1016/s0140-6736(12)61144-1

[2] Jin HL, Dong JC. Pathogenesis of idiopathic pulmonary fibrosis: From initial apoptosis of epithelial cells to lung remodeling. Chinese Medical Journal. 2011;**124**(24):4330-4338

[3] Leask A, Abraham DJ. TGF-beta signaling and the fibrotic response. The FASEB Journal. 2004;**18**(7):816-827. DOI: 10.1096/fj.03-1273rev

[4] Raghu G, Remy-Jardin M, Myers JL, Richeldi L, Ryerson CJ, Lederer DJ, et al. Diagnosis of idiopathic pulmonary fibrosis: An official ATS/ERS/JRS/ALAT clinical practice guideline. American Journal of Respiratory and Critical Care Medicine. 2018;**198**(5):e44-e68. DOI: 10.1164/rccm.201807-1255ST

[5] Winter J, Jung S, Keller S, Gregory RI, Diederichs S. Many roads to maturity: MicroRNA biogenesis pathways and their regulation. Nature Cell Biology. 2009;**11**(3):228-234. DOI: 10.1038/ncb0309-228

[6] Bushati N, Cohen SM. MicroRNA functions. Annual Review of Cell and Developmental Biology. 2007;**23**:175-205. DOI: 10.1146/annurev.cellbio.23.090506.123406

[7] Leung AK, Sharp PA. MicroRNA functions in stress responses. Molecular Cell. 2010;**40**(2):205-215. DOI: 10.1016/j.molcel.2010.09.027

[8] O'Connell RM, Rao DS, Baltimore D. MicroRNA regulation of inflammatory responses. Annual Review of Immunology. 2012;**30**:295-312. DOI: 10.1146/annurev-immunol-020711-075013

[9] Medina PP, Nolde M, Slack FJ. OncomiR addiction in an in vivo model of microRNA-21-induced pre-B-cell lymphoma. Nature. 2010;**467**(7311):86-90. DOI: 10.1038/nature09284

[10] Chowdhury SR, Reimer A, Sharan M, Kozjak-Pavlovic V, Eulalio A, Prusty BK, et al. Chlamydia preserves the mitochondrial network necessary for replication via microRNA-dependent inhibition of fission. The Journal of Cell Biology. 2017;**216**(4):1071-1089. DOI: 10.1083/jcb.201608063

[11] Li XX, Liu YM, Li YJ, Xie N, Yan YF, Chi YL, et al. High glucose concentration induces endothelial cell proliferation by regulating cyclin-D2-related miR-98. Journal of Cellular and Molecular Medicine. 2016;**20**(6):1159-1169. DOI: 10.1111/jcmm.12765

[12] Takagi K, Yamakuchi M, Matsuyama T, Kondo K, Uchida A, Misono S, et al. IL-13 enhances mesenchymal transition of pulmonary artery endothelial cells via down-regulation of miR-424/503 in vitro. Cellular Signalling. 2018;**42**:270-280. DOI: 10.1016/j.cellsig.2017.10.019

[13] Kim J, Hwangbo C, Hu X, Kang Y, Papangeli I, Mehrotra D, et al. Restoration of impaired endothelial myocyte enhancer factor 2 function rescues pulmonary arterial hypertension. Circulation. 2015;**131**(2):190-199. DOI: 10.1161/circulationaha.114.013339

[14] Lu TX, Munitz A, Rothenberg ME. MicroRNA-21 is up-regulated in allergic airway inflammation and regulates IL-12p35 expression. Journal of Immunology. 2009;**182**(8):4994-5002. DOI: 10.4049/jimmunol.0803560

[15] Mattes J, Collison A, Plank M, Phipps S, Foster PS. Antagonism

of microRNA-126 suppresses the effector function of TH2 cells and the development of allergic airways disease. Proceedings of the National Academy of Sciences of the United States of America. 2009;**106**(44):18704-18709. DOI: 10.1073/pnas.0905063106

[16] Collison A, Mattes J, Plank M, Foster PS. Inhibition of house dust mite-induced allergic airways disease by antagonism of microRNA-145 is comparable to glucocorticoid treatment. The Journal of Allergy and Clinical Immunology. 2011;**128**(1):160-7e4. DOI: 10.1016/j.jaci.2011.04.005

[17] Qin HB, Xu B, Mei JJ, Li D, Liu JJ, Zhao DY, et al. Inhibition of miRNA-221 suppresses the airway inflammation in asthma. Inflammation. 2012;**35**(4):1595-1599. DOI: 10.1007/s10753-012-9474-1

[18] Pandit KV, Corcoran D, Yousef H, Yarlagadda M, Tzouvelekis A, Gibson KF, et al. Inhibition and role of let-7d in idiopathic pulmonary fibrosis. American Journal of Respiratory and Critical Care Medicine. 2010;**182**(2):220-229. DOI: 10.1164/rccm.200911-1698OC

[19] Liu G, Friggeri A, Yang Y, Milosevic J, Ding Q, Thannickal VJ, et al. miR-21 mediates fibrogenic activation of pulmonary fibroblasts and lung fibrosis. The Journal of Experimental Medicine. 2010;**207**(8):1589-1597. DOI: 10.1084/jem.20100035

[20] Cushing L, Kuang PP, Qian J, Shao F, Wu J, Little F, et al. miR-29 is a major regulator of genes associated with pulmonary fibrosis. American Journal of Respiratory Cell and Molecular Biology. 2011;**45**(2):287-294. DOI: 10.1165/rcmb.2010-0323OC

[21] Pottier N, Maurin T, Chevalier B, Puissegur MP, Lebrigand K, Robbe-Sermesant K, et al. Identification of keratinocyte growth factor as a target of microRNA-155 in lung fibroblasts: Implication in epithelial-mesenchymal interactions. PLoS One. 2009;**4**(8):e6718. DOI: 10.1371/journal.pone.0006718

[22] Oak SR, Murray L, Herath A, Sleeman M, Anderson I, Joshi AD, et al. A micro RNA processing defect in rapidly progressing idiopathic pulmonary fibrosis. PLoS One. 2011;**6**(6):e21253. DOI: 10.1371/journal.pone.0021253

[23] Zhou J, Xu Q, Zhang Q, Wang Z, Guan S. A novel molecular mechanism of microRNA-21 inducing pulmonary fibrosis and human pulmonary fibroblast extracellular matrix through transforming growth factor beta1-mediated SMADs activation. Journal of Cellular Biochemistry. 2018;**119**(9):7834-7843. DOI: 10.1002/jcb.27185

[24] Huang C, Xiao X, Yang Y, Mishra A, Liang Y, Zeng X, et al. MicroRNA-101 attenuates pulmonary fibrosis by inhibiting fibroblast proliferation and activation. The Journal of Biological Chemistry. 2017;**292**(40):16420-16439. DOI: 10.1074/jbc.M117.805747

[25] Zhang S, Liu H, Liu Y, Zhang J, Li H, Liu W, et al. miR-30a as potential therapeutics by targeting TET1 through regulation of Drp-1 promoter hydroxymethylation in idiopathic pulmonary fibrosis. International Journal of Molecular Sciences. 2017;**18**(3). DOI: 10.3390/ijms18030633

[26] Li P, Zhao GQ, Chen TF, Chang JX, Wang HQ, Chen SS, et al. Serum miR-21 and miR-155 expression in idiopathic pulmonary fibrosis. The Journal of Asthma. 2013;**50**(9):960-964. DOI: 10.3109/02770903.2013.822080

[27] Njock MS, Guiot J, Henket MA, Nivelles O, Thiry M, Dequiedt F, et al. Sputum exosomes: Promising biomarkers for idiopathic pulmonary

fibrosis. Thorax. 2018. DOI: 10.1136/thoraxjnl-2018-211897

[28] Bibaki E, Tsitoura E, Vasarmidi E, Margaritopoulos G, Trachalaki A, Koutoulaki C, et al. miR-185 and miR-29a are similarly expressed in the bronchoalveolar lavage cells in IPF and lung cancer but common targets DNMT1 and COL1A1 show disease specific patterns. Molecular Medicine Reports. 2018;**17**(5):7105-7112. DOI: 10.3892/mmr.2018.8778

[29] Tsitoura E, Wells AU, Karagiannis K, Lasithiotaki I, Vasarmidi E, Bibaki E, et al. miR-185/AKT and miR-29a/collagen 1a pathways are activated in IPF BAL cells. Oncotarget. 2016;**7**(46):74569-74581. DOI: 10.18632/oncotarget.12740

[30] Dai WJ, Qiu J, Sun J, Ma CL, Huang N, Jiang Y, et al. Downregulation of microRNA-9 reduces inflammatory response and fibroblast proliferation in mice with idiopathic pulmonary fibrosis through the ANO1-mediated TGF-beta-Smad3 pathway. Journal of Cellular Physiology. 2019:**234**(3):2552-2565. DOI: 10.1002/jcp.26961

[31] Liang H, Liu S, Chen Y, Bai X, Liu L, Dong Y, et al. miR-26a suppresses EMT by disrupting the Lin28B/let-7d axis: Potential cross-talks among miRNAs in IPF. Journal of Molecular Medicine (Berlin). 2016;**94**(6):655-665. DOI: 10.1007/s00109-016-1381-8

[32] Wang Y, Liang Y, Luo J, Nie J, Yin H, Chen Q , et al. XIST/miR-139 axis regulates bleomycin (BLM)-induced extracellular matrix (ECM) and pulmonary fibrosis through beta-catenin. Oncotarget. 2017;**8**(39):65359-65369. DOI: 10.18632/oncotarget.18310

[33] Yang S, Banerjee S, de Freitas A, Sanders YY, Ding Q , Matalon S, et al. Participation of miR-200 in pulmonary fibrosis. The American Journal of Pathology. 2012;**180**(2):484-493. DOI: 10.1016/j.ajpath.2011.10.005

[34] Das S, Kumar M, Negi V, Pattnaik B, Prakash YS, Agrawal A, et al. MicroRNA-326 regulates profibrotic functions of transforming growth factor-beta in pulmonary fibrosis. American Journal of Respiratory Cell and Molecular Biology. 2014;**50**(5):882-892. DOI: 10.1165/rcmb.2013-0195OC

[35] Liu B, Li R, Zhang J, Meng C, Zhang J, Song X, et al. MicroRNA-708-3p as a potential therapeutic target via the ADAM17-GATA/STAT3 axis in idiopathic pulmonary fibrosis. Experimental and Molecular Medicine. 2018;**50**(3):e465. DOI: 10.1038/emm.2017.311

[36] Yan W, Wu Q , Yao W, Li Y, Liu Y, Yuan J, et al. miR-503 modulates epithelial-mesenchymal transition in silica-induced pulmonary fibrosis by targeting PI3K p85 and is sponged by lncRNA MALAT1. Scientific Reports. 2017;**7**(1):11313. DOI: 10.1038/s41598-017-11904-8

[37] Wu Q , Han L, Yan W, Ji X, Han R, Yang J, et al. miR-489 inhibits silica-induced pulmonary fibrosis by targeting MyD88 and Smad3 and is negatively regulated by lncRNA CHRF. Scientific Reports. 2016;**6**:30921. DOI: 10.1038/srep30921

[38] Liang H, Xu C, Pan Z, Zhang Y, Xu Z, Chen Y, et al. The antifibrotic effects and mechanisms of microRNA-26a action in idiopathic pulmonary fibrosis. Molecular Therapy. 2014;**22**(6):1122-1133. DOI: 10.1038/mt.2014.42

[39] Selman M, Pardo A. Role of epithelial cells in idiopathic pulmonary fibrosis: From innocent targets to serial killers. Proceedings of the American Thoracic Society. 2006;**3**(4):364-372. DOI: 10.1513/pats.200601-003TK

[40] Tanjore H, Lawson WE, Blackwell TS. Endoplasmic reticulum stress as

a pro-fibrotic stimulus. Biochimica et Biophysica Acta. 2013;**1832**(7):940-947. DOI: 10.1016/j.bbadis.2012.11.011

[41] Scotton CJ, Chambers RC. Molecular targets in pulmonary fibrosis: The myofibroblast in focus. Chest. 2007;**132**(4):1311-1321. DOI: 10.1378/chest.06-2568

[42] Bellaye PS, Kolb M. Why do patients get idiopathic pulmonary fibrosis? Current concepts in the pathogenesis of pulmonary fibrosis. BMC Medicine. 2015;**13**:176. DOI: 10.1186/s12916-015-0412-6

[43] Heath D, Gillund TD, Kay JM, Hawkins CF. Pulmonary vascular disease in honeycomb lung. The Journal of Pathology and Bacteriology. 1968;**95**(2):423-430. DOI: 10.1002/path.1700950212

[44] Blanco I, Ribas J, Xaubet A, Gomez FP, Roca J, Rodriguez-Roisin R, et al. Effects of inhaled nitric oxide at rest and during exercise in idiopathic pulmonary fibrosis. Journal of Applied Physiology (Bethesda, Md: 1985). 2011;**110**(3):638-645. DOI: 10.1152/japplphysiol.01104.2010

[45] Hashimoto N, Phan SH, Imaizumi K, Matsuo M, Nakashima H, Kawabe T, et al. Endothelial-mesenchymal transition in bleomycin-induced pulmonary fibrosis. American Journal of Respiratory Cell and Molecular Biology. 2010;**43**(2):161-172. DOI: 10.1165/rcmb.2009-0031OC

[46] Yeager ME, Frid MG, Stenmark KR. Progenitor cells in pulmonary vascular remodeling. Pulmonary Circulation. 2011;**1**(1):3-16. DOI: 10.4103/2045-8932.78095

[47] Song E, Ouyang N, Horbelt M, Antus B, Wang M, Exton MS. Influence of alternatively and classically activated macrophages on fibrogenic activities of human fibroblasts. Cellular Immunology. 2000;**204**(1):19-28. DOI: 10.1006/cimm.2000.1687

[48] Atabai K, Jame S, Azhar N, Kuo A, Lam M, McKleroy W, et al. Mfge8 diminishes the severity of tissue fibrosis in mice by binding and targeting collagen for uptake by macrophages. The Journal of Clinical Investigation. 2009;**119**(12):3713-3722. DOI: 10.1172/jci40053

[49] Murray PJ, Wynn TA. Protective and pathogenic functions of macrophage subsets. Nature Reviews. Immunology. 2011;**11**(11):723-737. DOI: 10.1038/nri3073

[50] Murray LA, Chen Q, Kramer MS, Hesson DP, Argentieri RL, Peng X, et al. TGF-beta driven lung fibrosis is macrophage dependent and blocked by Serum amyloid P. The International Journal of Biochemistry and Cell Biology. 2011;**43**(1):154-162. DOI: 10.1016/j.biocel.2010.10.013

[51] Murray LA, Rosada R, Moreira AP, Joshi A, Kramer MS, Hesson DP, et al. Serum amyloid P therapeutically attenuates murine bleomycin-induced pulmonary fibrosis via its effects on macrophages. PLoS One. 2010;**5**(3):e9683. DOI: 10.1371/journal.pone.0009683

[52] Gibbons MA, MacKinnon AC, Ramachandran P, Dhaliwal K, Duffin R, Phythian-Adams AT, et al. Ly6Chi monocytes direct alternatively activated profibrotic macrophage regulation of lung fibrosis. American Journal of Respiratory and Critical Care Medicine. 2011;**184**(5):569-581. DOI: 10.1164/rccm.201010-1719OC

[53] Rosas IO, Ren P, Avila NA, Chow CK, Franks TJ, Travis WD, et al. Early interstitial lung disease in familial pulmonary fibrosis. American Journal of Respiratory and Critical Care Medicine. 2007;**176**(7):698-705. DOI: 10.1164/rccm.200702-254OC

[54] Marchal-Somme J, Uzunhan Y, Marchand-Adam S, Kambouchner M, Valeyre D, Crestani B, et al. Dendritic cells accumulate in human fibrotic interstitial lung disease. American Journal of Respiratory and Critical Care Medicine. 2007;**176**(10):1007-1014. DOI: 10.1164/rccm.200609-1347OC

[55] Kotsianidis I, Nakou E, Bouchliou I, Tzouvelekis A, Spanoudakis E, Steiropoulos P, et al. Global impairment of CD4+CD25+FOXP3+ regulatory T cells in idiopathic pulmonary fibrosis. American Journal of Respiratory and Critical Care Medicine. 2009;**179**(12):1121-1130. DOI: 10.1164/rccm.200812-1936OC

[56] Jerome T, Laurie P, Louis B, Pierre C. Enjoy the silence: The story of let-7 microRNA and cancer. Current Genomics. 2007;**8**(4):229-233

[57] Lewis BP, Burge CB, Bartel DP. Conserved seed pairing, often flanked by adenosines, indicates that thousands of human genes are microRNA targets. Cell. 2005;**120**(1):15-20. DOI: 10.1016/j.cell.2004.12.035

[58] Rosas IO, Richards TJ, Konishi K, Zhang Y, Gibson K, Lokshin AE, et al. MMP1 and MMP7 as potential peripheral blood biomarkers in idiopathic pulmonary fibrosis. PLoS Medicine. 2008;**5**(4):e93. DOI: 10.1371/journal.pmed.0050093

[59] Liang H, Gu Y, Li T, Zhang Y, Huangfu L, Hu M, et al. Integrated analyses identify the involvement of microRNA-26a in epithelial-mesenchymal transition during idiopathic pulmonary fibrosis. Cell Death and Disease. 2014;**5**:e1238. DOI: 10.1038/cddis.2014.207

[60] Christoffersen NR, Silahtaroglu A, Orom UA, Kauppinen S, Lund AH. miR-200b mediates post-transcriptional repression of ZFHX1B. RNA. 2007;**13**(8):1172-1178. DOI: 10.1261/rna.586807

[61] Hurteau GJ, Carlson JA, Spivack SD, Brock GJ. Overexpression of the microRNA hsa-miR-200c leads to reduced expression of transcription factor 8 and increased expression of E-cadherin. Cancer Research. 2007;**67**(17):7972-7976. DOI: 10.1158/0008-5472.can-07-1058

[62] Spaderna S, Schmalhofer O, Hlubek F, Berx G, Eger A, Merkel S, et al. A transient, EMT-linked loss of basement membranes indicates metastasis and poor survival in colorectal cancer. Gastroenterology. 2006;**131**(3):830-840. DOI: 10.1053/j.gastro.2006.06.016

[63] Korpal M, Lee ES, Hu G, Kang Y. The miR-200 family inhibits epithelial-mesenchymal transition and cancer cell migration by direct targeting of E-cadherin transcriptional repressors ZEB1 and ZEB2. The Journal of Biological Chemistry. 2008;**283**(22):14910-14914. DOI: 10.1074/jbc.C800074200

[64] Kisseleva T, Brenner DA. Mechanisms of fibrogenesis. Experimental Biology and Medicine (Maywood, N.J.). 2008;**233**(2):109-122. DOI: 10.3181/0707-mr-190

[65] Stolzenburg LR, Wachtel S, Dang H, Harris A. miR-1343 attenuates pathways of fibrosis by targeting the TGF-beta receptors. The Biochemical Journal. 2016;**473**(3):245-256. DOI: 10.1042/bj20150821

[66] Pandit KV, Milosevic J, Kaminski N. MicroRNAs in idiopathic pulmonary fibrosis. Translational Research. 2011;**157**(4):191-199. DOI: 10.1016/j.trsl.2011.01.012

[67] Matsushima S, Ishiyama J. MicroRNA-29c regulates apoptosis sensitivity via modulation of the cell-surface death receptor, Fas, in lung fibroblasts. American Journal of Physiology. Lung Cellular and Molecular

Physiology. 2016;**311**(6):L1050-L1L61. DOI: 10.1152/ajplung.00252.2016

[68] Montgomery RL, Yu G, Latimer PA, Stack C, Robinson K, Dalby CM, et al. MicroRNA mimicry blocks pulmonary fibrosis. EMBO Molecular Medicine. 2014;**6**(10):1347-1356. DOI: 10.15252/emmm.201303604

[69] Senavirathna LK, Huang C, Yang X, Munteanu MC, Sathiaseelan R, Xu D, et al. Hypoxia induces pulmonary fibroblast proliferation through NFAT signaling. Scientific Reports. 2018;**8**(1):2709. DOI: 10.1038/s41598-018-21073-x

[70] Liang C, Zhu H, Xu Y, Huang L, Ma C, Deng W, et al. MicroRNA-153 negatively regulates the expression of amyloid precursor protein and amyloid precursor-like protein 2. Brain Research. 2012;**1455**:103-113. DOI: 10.1016/j.brainres.2011.10.051

[71] Xie T, Liang J, Guo R, Liu N, Noble PW, Jiang D. Comprehensive microRNA analysis in bleomycin-induced pulmonary fibrosis identifies multiple sites of molecular regulation. Physiological Genomics. 2011;**43**(9):479-487. DOI: 10.1152/physiolgenomics.00222.2010

[72] Liang C, Li X, Zhang L, Cui D, Quan X, Yang W. The anti-fibrotic effects of microRNA-153 by targeting TGFBR-2 in pulmonary fibrosis. Experimental and Molecular Pathology. 2015;**99**(2):279-285. DOI: 10.1016/j.yexmp.2015.07.011

[73] Milosevic J, Pandit K, Magister M, Rabinovich E, Ellwanger DC, Yu G, et al. Profibrotic role of miR-154 in pulmonary fibrosis. American Journal of Respiratory Cell and Molecular Biology. 2012;**47**(6):879-887. DOI: 10.1165/rcmb.2011-0377OC

[74] Kurowska-Stolarska M, Alivernini S, Ballantine LE, Asquith DL, Millar NL,

Gilchrist DS, et al. MicroRNA-155 as a proinflammatory regulator in clinical and experimental arthritis. Proceedings of the National Academy of Sciences of the United States of America. 2011;**108**(27):11193-11198. DOI: 10.1073/pnas.1019536108

[75] O'Connell RM, Rao DS, Chaudhuri AA, Boldin MP, Taganov KD, Nicoll J, et al. Sustained expression of microRNA-155 in hematopoietic stem cells causes a myeloproliferative disorder. The Journal of Experimental Medicine. 2008;**205**(3):585-594. DOI: 10.1084/jem.20072108

[76] Rodriguez A, Vigorito E, Clare S, Warren MV, Couttet P, Soond DR, et al. Requirement of bic/microRNA-155 for normal immune function. Science. 2007;**316**(5824):608-611. DOI: 10.1126/science.1139253

[77] Kurowska-Stolarska M, Hasoo MK, Welsh DJ, Stewart L, McIntyre D, Morton BE, et al. The role of microRNA-155/liver X receptor pathway in experimental and idiopathic pulmonary fibrosis. The Journal of Allergy and Clinical Immunology. 2017;**139**(6):1946-1956. DOI: 10.1016/j.jaci.2016.09.021

[78] Bodempudi V, Hergert P, Smith K, Xia H, Herrera J, Peterson M, et al. miR-210 promotes IPF fibroblast proliferation in response to hypoxia. American Journal of Physiology. Lung Cellular and Molecular Physiology. 2014;**307**(4):L283-L294. DOI: 10.1152/ajplung.00069.2014

[79] Patel NM, Lederer DJ, Borczuk AC, Kawut SM. Pulmonary hypertension in idiopathic pulmonary fibrosis. Chest. 2007;**132**(3):998-1006. DOI: 10.1378/chest.06-3087

[80] Xu X, Tan X, Tampe B, Sanchez E, Zeisberg M, Zeisberg EM. Snail is a direct target of hypoxia-inducible factor 1alpha (HIF1alpha) in hypoxia-induced

endothelial to mesenchymal transition of human coronary endothelial cells. The Journal of Biological Chemistry. 2015;**290**(27):16653-16664. DOI: 10.1074/jbc.M115.636944

[81] Saharinen P, Kerkela K, Ekman N, Marron M, Brindle N, Lee GM, et al. Multiple angiopoietin recombinant proteins activate the Tie1 receptor tyrosine kinase and promote its interaction with Tie2. The Journal of Cell Biology. 2005;**169**(2):239-243. DOI: 10.1083/jcb.200411105

[82] Kugathasan L, Ray JB, Deng Y, Rezaei E, Dumont DJ, Stewart DJ. The angiopoietin-1-Tie2 pathway prevents rather than promotes pulmonary arterial hypertension in transgenic mice. The Journal of Experimental Medicine. 2009;**206**(10):2221-2234. DOI: 10.1084/jem.20090389

[83] Yuan HT, Venkatesha S, Chan B, Deutsch U, Mammoto T, Sukhatme VP, et al. Activation of the orphan endothelial receptor Tie1 modifies Tie2-mediated intracellular signaling and cell survival. The FASEB Journal. 2007;**21**(12):3171-3183. DOI: 10.1096/fj.07-8487com

[84] Liu XB, Jiang J, Gui C, Hu XY, Xiang MX, Wang JA. Angiopoietin-1 protects mesenchymal stem cells against serum deprivation and hypoxia-induced apoptosis through the PI3K/Akt pathway. Acta Pharmacologica Sinica. 2008;**29**(7):815-822. DOI: 10.1111/j.1745-7254.2008.00811.x

[85] Humbert M, Morrell NW, Archer SL, Stenmark KR, MR ML, Lang IM, et al. Cellular and molecular pathobiology of pulmonary arterial hypertension. Journal of the American College of Cardiology. 2004;**43**(12 Suppl S):13S-24S. DOI: 10.1016/j.jacc.2004.02.029

[86] Wang P, Xu J, Hou Z, Wang F, Song Y, Wang J, et al. miRNA-34a promotes

proliferation of human pulmonary artery smooth muscle cells by targeting PDGFRA. Cell Proliferation. 2016;**49**(4):484-493. DOI: 10.1111/cpr.12265

[87] Syed M, Das P, Pawar A, Aghai ZH, Kaskinen A, Zhuang ZW, et al. Hyperoxia causes miR-34a-mediated injury via angiopoietin-1 in neonatal lungs. Nature Communications. 2017;**8**(1):1173. DOI: 10.1038/s41467-017-01349-y

[88] Qu Y, Zhang G, Ji Y, Zhua H, Lv C, Jiang W. Protective role of gambogic acid in experimental pulmonary fibrosis in vitro and in vivo. Phytomedicine. 2016;**23**(4):350-358. DOI: 10.1016/j.phymed.2016.01.011

[89] Gordon S, Martinez FO. Alternative activation of macrophages: Mechanism and functions. Immunity. 2010;**32**(5):593-604. DOI: 10.1016/j.immuni.2010.05.007

[90] Su S, Liu Q , Chen J, Chen J, Chen F, He C, et al. A positive feedback loop between mesenchymal-like cancer cells and macrophages is essential to breast cancer metastasis. Cancer Cell. 2014;**25**(5):605-620. DOI: 10.1016/j.ccr.2014.03.021

[91] Fichtner-Feigl S, Strober W, Kawakami K, Puri RK, Kitani A. IL-13 signaling through the IL-13alpha2 receptor is involved in induction of TGF-beta1 production and fibrosis. Nature Medicine. 2006;**12**(1):99-106. DOI: 10.1038/nm1332

[92] Prasse A, Pechkovsky DV, Toews GB, Jungraithmayr W, Kollert F, Goldmann T, et al. A vicious circle of alveolar macrophages and fibroblasts perpetuates pulmonary fibrosis via CCL18. American Journal of Respiratory and Critical Care Medicine. 2006;**173**(7):781-792. DOI: 10.1164/rccm.200509-1518OC

[93] Sica A, Mantovani A. Macrophage plasticity and polarization: In vivo veritas. The Journal of Clinical Investigation. 2012;**122**(3):787-795. DOI: 10.1172/jci59643

[94] Su S, Zhao Q , He C, Huang D, Liu J, Chen F, et al. miR-142-5p and miR-130a-3p are regulated by IL-4 and IL-13 and control profibrogenic macrophage program. Nature Communications. 2015;**6**:8523. DOI: 10.1038/ncomms9523

[95] Nakashima T, Yokoyama A, Onari Y, Shoda H, Haruta Y, Hattori N, et al. Suppressor of cytokine signaling 1 inhibits pulmonary inflammation and fibrosis. The Journal of Allergy and Clinical Immunology. 2008;**121**(5):1269-1276. DOI: 10.1016/j.jaci.2008.02.003

[96] Lei GS, Kline HL, Lee CH, Wilkes DS, Zhang C. Regulation of collagen V expression and epithelial-mesenchymal transition by miR-185 and miR-186 during idiopathic pulmonary fibrosis. The American Journal of Pathology. 2016;**186**(9):2310-2316. DOI: 10.1016/j.ajpath.2016.04.015

[97] Qadir XV, Han C, Lu D, Zhang J, Wu T. miR-185 inhibits hepatocellular carcinoma growth by targeting the DNMT1/PTEN/Akt pathway. The American Journal of Pathology. 2014;**184**(8):2355-2364. DOI: 10.1016/j.ajpath.2014.05.004

[98] Takahashi Y, Forrest AR, Maeno E, Hashimoto T, Daub CO, Yasuda J. miR-107 and MiR-185 can induce cell cycle arrest in human non small cell lung cancer cell lines. PLoS One. 2009;**4**(8):e6677. DOI: 10.1371/journal.pone.0006677

[99] Betensley A, Sharif R, Karamichos D. A systematic review of the role of dysfunctional wound healing in the pathogenesis and treatment of idiopathic pulmonary fibrosis. Journal of Clinical Medicine. 2016;**6**(1). DOI: 10.3390/jcm6010002

[100] Daniel E, Roff A, Hsu MH, Panganiban R, Lambert K, Ishmael F. Effects of allergic stimulation and glucocorticoids on miR-155 in CD4(+) T-cells. American Journal of Clinical and Experimental Immunology. 2018;**7**(4):57-66

[101] Wang J, Yang L, Wang L, Yang Y, Wang Y. Forkhead box p3 controls progression of oral lichen planus by regulating microRNA-146a. Journal of Cellular Biochemistry. 2018;**119**(11):8862-8871. DOI: 10.1002/jcb.27139

Chapter 3

Lung Transplantation: A Final Option for End-Stage Interstitial Lung Diseases

Mohammed Fakhro and Sandra Lindstedt

Abstract

Lung transplantation (LTx) is an established, well-recognized medical intervention for treating patients with an end-stage irreversible pulmonary disease. Such diseases include interstitial lung disease (ILD), where other standard medical options often have been proven as insufficient. Post-operative survival after LTx depends on various factors such as the general and organ-specific recipient status in addition to donor organ condition and operative technique. The prolonged survival rates obtained during the 1980s and 1990s have established LTx in the medical field. Reflecting the improvements made in the field of organ preservation, operative technique, immunosuppressants, recipient and donor organ selection and prophylactic as well as direct treatment in the wide spectrum of possible infections in the recipient. Despite LTx being the golden standard for treating end-stage irreversible ILD, with idiopathic pulmonary fibrosis (IPF) as the most common cause, post-operative outcome is greatly hampered compared to the outcome of other patient categories within LTx. This chapter will provide insight in the outcome of ILD and subsequently IFP after LTx.

Keywords: lung, transplantation, post-operative outcome, long-term follow-up, interstitial lung diseases, interstitial pulmonary fibrosis

1. Introduction

Lung transplantation (LTx) is a known medical intervention for irreversible/end stage lung diseases, where standard medical treatment has been proven to be insufficient, such as patients with end-stage interstitial lung disease (ILD) [1].

Other medical interventions for ILD are restricted to corticosteroids and cytotoxic pharmaceuticals with reports showing up to 90% of this patient group as non-responsive to pharmaceuticals [2–4].

Idiopathic pulmonary fibrosis (IPF) was the diagnosis for the first LTx among long-term surviving patients that was successful, performed in 1983 at Toronto. IPF is regularly found in recipients that have undertaken LTx for end-stage pulmonary disease [5, 6].

ILD is problematic to treat and often with poor prognosis. Especially IPF that has an outcome that is among the poorest in ILD, with a median survival of up to 3 years after time of diagnosis [7]. As IPF is an incurable disease, it has additionally been reported that if untreated presents with a 5-year survival of 30–50% [3, 4, 8, 9].

Post-operative outcome of LTx rests on several aspects, for instance general and organ specific patient status, donor graft status and operative method. The extended survival estimates attained in the 80s and 90s most probably mirror developments in graft preservation, operative practice, immunosuppressive agents, recipient/donor graft selection, and prophylactic therapies of opportunistic infections in the recipient [10].

These progressions in averting early adverse events have permitted a wider incline of indications in LTx with a steady liberalization of donor criteria. This has provided a general growth in LTx, although this quantity is yet to date constrained by donor organ scarcity. Even though numerous difficulties after LTx persist (e.g., opportunistic infections, graft rejection, and pathological relapse in the donor graft), LTx is the definitive option for candidates with advanced loss of pulmonary function triggered by advanced IPF. The quantity of LTxs achieved is principally restricted by the low availability of donor organs [11]. Survival is meager for IPF recipients when compared to basically all other pulmonary disease groups.

2. Patients and methods

2.1 Transplant procedure

Five types of Tx procedures are normally presented:

- Single lung transplantation (SLTx)

- Double lung transplantation (DLTx)

- Heart-lung transplantation (HLTx)

- Cadaveric lobar transplants (CLTx)

- Transplantation of lobes from living related donors

Throughout the course of listing a patient with ILD for LTx, the patient's indication for Tx as well as preference for DLTx or SLTx, comorbidities, operative risk, blood type, and donor specific antibodies are investigated beforehand. Both SLTx and DLTx are achieved in recipients with IPF and discussion is present yet to date whether SLTx or DLTx is the superior alternative in this specific group [12].

2.2 Recipient selection

Recipients are selected differently from center to center. In the Lund university model as an example, recipients can be selected according to the guidelines by the consensus report from the Pulmonary Scientific Council of the International Society for Heart and Lung Transplantation [13]. Inclusion norms are often candidates diagnosed with chronic lung pathology who are non-responsive to other medical treatment. LTx candidates characteristically have a life expectancy of less than 18 months and are often dependent on additional oxygen present and are often physically restricted. Before entering a LTx programme, candidates usually undergo a clinical investigation that can consist of following:

a. evaluation of kidney function (GFR) by iohexol clearance;

b. immunological screening;

c. microbiological screening;

d. hematological and biochemical laboratory testing;

e. virologic screening;

f. dental examination;

g. densitometry;

h. stress test with arterial blood gas, lung scintigraphy and spirometry;

i. Doppler of the carotid arteries (>50 years);

j. CT scan of the chest and abdomen;

k. echocardiogram;

l. coronary angiography of coronary blood vessels; and

m. 24 hours pH evaluation, sometimes followed by gastroscopy.

Patients are often reviewed by a multidisciplinary team before accepted for LTx. Recipient/donor matching can be based on ABO blood type and graft size.

The United Network for Organ Sharing (UNOS) has implemented a lung allocation score (LAS) in the United States. The LAS is a resolve to classify patients in most need of a LTx. The LAS is designed by means of numerous evaluations of a patient's status that approximate outcome and predicting the period of survival with or without a LTx. Application of the LAS gave rise to an improved quantity of IPF patients getting a LTx as IPF developed into the biggest and most common major indication to accept a LTx in 2007 in the United States [14]. In 2011, patients with IPF yielded the biggest proportion (46%) of candidates on the LTx wait-list in the US.

Diverse clinical methods are utilized to properly rank for LTx. Biopsy results are supportive in deciding the precise diagnosis for IPF [13, 15]. Conventionally, numerous clinicians have utilized lung function tests to decide the appropriate period of listing a ILD/IPF patient for LTx, with a report that lung function testing through diffusion pulmonary function for CO < 39% may predict early mortality [16] in addition to 6-minute walk test (6MWT) that can predict early mortality [17]. Radiologic findings are of great value in sorting ILD patients in terms of hazard. High-resolution computed tomography has shown that a greater grade of fibrosis forecasts greater risk for death [18, 19].

Patients with IPF although placed on the waiting list for LTx, such a patient is still exposed to great hazard. In history, IPF patients have the highest waiting list mortality estimates of all candidates for LTx [20, 21]. Before the LAS, candidates with IPF showed a waiting list mortality between 28 and 47% with other recipient groups presenting a waiting-list mortality at only 15% [2, 3, 22]. Due to the great risk in mortality as well as morbidity on the waiting list, it is of great interest to investigate methods to optimize this process. 15-step oximetry test, 6MWT as well as the quantity of oxygen that the IPF recipient is dependent on have all a role to play in reflecting the risk of mortality on the waiting list [22–24]. Further improvements are needed in maintaining the well-being of this patient group in waiting for a LTx.

2.3 Donor organ selection

Matching a donor lung with a recipient can be grounded on donor/recipient height and even pulmonary volume from chest radiographs [25, 26]. The optimal grade of fit is not known and the association between donor and recipient do not have to be a perfect match, but a close match is favored in terms of size [27].

"Ideal donor criteria" are often thought of as age < 55 years, normal chest X-ray, PaO_2/FiO_2 > 300 mmHg at five PEEP, <20 pack year smoking history, lack of chest trauma and lack of aspiration/sepsis [27, 28].

2.4 Immunosuppression

Maintenance of immunoregulation depends on the center and region. With the Lund University model as an example, it has remained more or less the same during the LTx programmes inception, based on a practice of cyclosporine, corticosteroids and azathioprine or mykofenolatmofetil as a lifelong routine.

2.5 Antimicrobial and infection prophylaxis

LTx patients are at increased hazard for infectious difficulties because of subsequent features:

- High level of immunosuppression to prevent rejection

- Adversative consequences from Tx on the lung host defenses

- Persistent environmental interaction permitting microbiological agents direct admission into the graft

The probability and category of infection differs with the degree of recipient immunosuppression, timing since LTx, variety and period of anti-microbial prophylaxis in addition to the local center and regional microbiology. The most common type presented in LTx recipients are bacterial pneumonia [29, 30].

Prophylactic administration of broad-spectrum antibiotics such as carbapenem are preferred until cultures can be available and then initiate target treatment for specific infection. Antiviral therapy may be directed against CMV for recipients with positive CMV serology. Preoperative screening for CMV is performed routinely in recipients/donors. Antifungal prophylaxis may include low-dose fluconazole for Candida and sulfametoxazol/trimethoprim for *Pneumocystis carinii*. Broad-spectrum antibiotics with colistin may be utilized for Pseudomonas if present.

2.6 Follow-up

Routine follow-up after LTx is intended to avert complications or to distinguish them as soon as possible. While follow-up is most rigorous during the first year after LTx, it is necessary to proceed with a lifetime of follow-up of the LTx recipient. Pulmonary function progressively advances and typically scopes a plateau by the end of year 1 after LTx [31, 32].

The practices include:

- Follow-up with a (trained) nurse coordinator

- Check-ups by a pneumonologist

- Chest X-ray

- Spirometry

- (Bronchoscopy)

- Selected hematological testing to supervise the immunosuppressive serum levels

There are also possibilities for the LTx recipient to be undergo follow-up from the home, such as daily home spirometry. This form of monitoring has been associated with earlier detection of chronic forms of rejection [33–37].

3. Outcomes after LTx

3.1 Survival

Outcome after LTx can be evaluated founded on numerous different measures: survival, quality of life, physiologic changes and cost benefit [38, 39]. Survival is feasibly the most objective calculation of outcome. The International Society for Heart and Lung Transplantation (ISHLT) has created a registry of survival estimates from international data that have become a benchmark for the field [40, 41]. According to the 2017 ISHLT registry report, the median survival for all adult LTx recipients is 6 years [38]. Nevertheless, it is uncertain if survival benefit is primarily connected to the type of procedure or the underlying LTx patient's features that does the impact. A report that assessed the influence of patient age and procedure on the survival outcome of patients with IPF showed that SLTx recipients younger than 60 years displayed a survival benefit over DLTx in the same age category [6].

The influence of the diagnostic type of recipient on survival after LTx has been studied expansively [38, 42, 43]. The primary major indication is habitually connected to age. Furthermore, specific diagnostic groups have a greater hazard of complications during LTx and primary graft dysfunction (PGD). Nevertheless, patients with COPD have the most superior first-year survival but then again a worse 10-year survival compared to other recipient groups such as pulmonary hypertension, sarcoidosis, and alpha-1 antitrypsin deficiency patients [38]. Those with IPF have the lowest 10-year outcome when compared to all other diagnostic groups.

Multiple report that have studied the post-LTx survival for IPF patients showed that 1-year survival range from 68 to 80%, 3-year survival from 50 to 61% and 5-year survival between 32 and 59%, with earlier LTx periods even tend to have worse outcome than recent LTxs performed [44–48]. There are various reports in post-LTx survival from monocentric data from Europe, North America as well as Brazil and Australia that show corresponding survival data for 1-year survival data ranging between 25 and 87% while 5-year survival has showed between 33 and 63% [22, 49–58].

3.2 DLTx versus SLTx

SLTx was the typical Tx type for recipients with IPF for several years and survival outcomes were analogous to other diagnostic groups within LTx [2, 5, 6, 22]. Though, a major proportion of IPF recipients are presently undergoing DLTx [59–61].

In 2011, almost half of all IPF patients where DLTxs while the other half where almost entirely SLTxs [62]. More than 60% of LTxs in 2014 for IPF recipients was DLTx while in 1991 this number was only 15% [60]. This alteration in trend is not entirely clear but it has been proposed that probable factors are better operative technique in addition to improved pulmonary function and survival for DLTx.

IPF patients that underwent DLTx has shown significantly better survival for DLTx versus SLTx, where survival has improved for DLTx patients with IPF compared to SLTx patients in this patient category [63]. Especially if IPF patients manage to survive beyond the 10-year mark, with attributed survival benefits in DLTx [64]. However it has also been reported that IPF patients that underwent DLTx do have an increased mortality risk in the early postoperative period [47]. In addition, when adjusting for risk factors in such analyses for DLTx vs. SLTx among IPF patients, no difference in outcome has been shown [65]. Other single centers such as from the US and Australia and data from the ISHLT from the period of 1994 to 2004 showed no difference in outcome regarding DLTx vs. SLTx for IPF patients [53, 66–68]. Interestingly, European centers has been able to show in contrast from the literature that SLTx has the ability to yield survival benefit for IPF patients than DLTx [69].

Living donor lobar LTx has been proposed as an option for LTx candidates with end-stage IPF with low probability to survive the entire period on the waiting list for standard donor LTx [70].

3.3 Ventilator support, intensive care and postoperative stay

Few studies have reported data on the early period in hospital stay post-LTx. One single center in Sweden however has reported ventilator support, intensive care unit stay and overall post-operative stay until discharge for all types of LTx recipients including IPF recipients [71]. This report showed that the median time for ventilator support after LTx was 2 days while for IPF patients that required almost 3 days. The same pattern followed for intensive care unit time after LTx, showing a median of over 6 days for all recipients while PF patients had a median of 8 days. Finally, the total time of hospital stay after LTx was a median of 43 days in all recipients while IPF patients had one of the longest at 46 days.

The studies that report post-LTx in hospital time and need of medical resources suggest that LTx in IPF patients has been associated with substantial resource use.

3.4 Cause of death and complications

Among IPF patients who underwent a LTx in the United States (1987–2009), the principal cause of death was infection or sepsis causing almost a quarter of the deaths of IPF recipients [2, 22, 47, 50, 55, 65, 68, 72, 73], followed by bronchiolitis obliterans syndrome (BOS)/chronic rejection [74].

As infection is the number one cause regarding complications, others causes include hemodynamic instability, kidney failure, myopathy, bleeding, and reoperation [75]. Almost a tenth of all LTx recipients may experience airway complications [76]. Malignancy is a long-term complication that almost a third of IPF patients may experience at 10 years after LTx [77]. In addition it is more common with lung embolisms in IPF patients with over a quarter of all patients in this category [49].

3.5 Rejection

PGD, a form of acute rejection is a severe complication that is a risk for all LTx recipients which include ILD patients. The background for this pathology depends on several factors though ischemia-reperfusion injury is assumed to be the main instrument of this pathology [78]. The incidence has been reported to be between 10 and 25% [78, 79]. Nonetheless, PGD in ILD patients are significantly more associated with worse mortality in the early outcome, whilst in the long-term is has been associated with increased risk of a form of chronic rejection as BOS [80]. Despite pulmonary hypertension recipients having a higher incidence of ischemia-reperfusion injury, recipients with IPF have a higher probability of experiencing ischemia-reperfusion injury than COPD patients, putting them at greater hazard of experiencing PGD [81].

BOS, a form of chronic lung allograft dysfunction, is the biggest factor hampering long-term outcome. Regrettably, it is likewise a common obstacle in LTx, where LTx recipients in general experience an incidence of almost 30% after 2 years and three quarters of recipients experience this pathology after 10 years [77, 82]. Recipients with IPF have a greater hazard of contracting PGD and therefore a greater hazard of BOS, where it is proposed that this patient group have steeper deterioration in lung function and greater risk of mortality than recipients without IPF that has been exposed to BOS [83, 84].

4. Conclusions

LTx is a well-known treatment strategy for an extensive number of irreversible end-stage pulmonary disease, including ILD with focus on IPF. There is yet to date a great gap among patients that is qualified and patients that are admitted for a LTx. IPF patients have a greater mortality on the waiting list versus other major indications. A great share of IPF patients decease before the possibility of undergoing LTx. This makes it important to prioritize this patient population for LTx as the need is unfortunately not met. IPF patients have been linked to greater risk of complications than other patient groups in parameters such as time in the intensive care unit, time in mechanical ventilator and in hospital time. It is still not entirely clear whether a SLTx or a DLTx is of greatest benefit to a IPF patient. The most recent trend has been in favor for DLTx rather than SLTx. It has been suggested that the increased survival in IPF patients is due to DLTx while on the other hand the data is conflicting. It is possible that a more accurate survival benefit is resulted among different subcategories of IPF candidates whilst on the other hand certain IPF candidates may not yield any survival benefit at all from a DLTx where greater understanding is required.

The application of the LAS has reduced the time on the waiting list and improved survival by yielding precedence for patients that are in the greatest need for a LTx. The implementation of the LAS gave rise to the IPF patient category to even surpass COPD as the greatest indication to undergo LTx. However, carrying out LTx in candidates with a greater LAS score does result in more extensive use of medical resources.

There is no curative treatment for IPF patients with a miserable prognosis. Up-to-date strategies for the inclusion of LTx candidates endorse that suitable IPF patients ought to be recruited for LTx at the earliest. IPF recipients show the worst outcome of all LTx patients in addition to the donor pool being hampered by the scarcity of donor organs. It is therefore essential that qualified ILD patients and above all IPF patients get selected for LTx in order to attain favorable long-term outcomes.

Conflict of interest

The authors declare that they have no competing interests.

Declarations

None declared.

Acronyms and abbreviations

LTx	lung transplantation
ILD	interstitial lung disease
IPF	idiopathic pulmonary fibrosis
SLTx	single lung transplantation
DLTx	double lung transplantation
HLTx	heart-lung transplantation
CLTx	cadaveric lobar transplants
UNOS	The United Network for Organ Sharing
LAS	lung allocation score
6MWT	6-minute walk test
ISHLT	The International Society for Heart and Lung Transplantation
PGD	primary graft dysfunction
BOS	bronchiolitis obliterans syndrome

Author details

Mohammed Fakhro and Sandra Lindstedt*
Department of Cardiothoracic Surgery, Skåne University Hospital, Lund University, Lund, Sweden

*Address all correspondence to: sandra.lindstedt_ingemansson@med.lu.se

IntechOpen

References

[1] Van Trigt P, Davis RD, Shaeffer GS, Gaynor JW, Landolfo KP, Higginbotham MB, et al. Survival benefits of heart and lung transplantation. Annals of Surgery. 1996;**223**:576-584

[2] Meyers BF, Lynch JP, Trulock EP, Guthrie T, Cooper JD, Patterson GA. Single versus bilateral lung transplantation for idiopathic pulmonary fibrosis: A ten-year institutional experience. The Journal of Thoracic and Cardiovascular Surgery. 2000;**120**:99-107

[3] Sulica R, Teirstein A, Padilla ML. Lung transplantation in interstitial lung disease. Current Opinion in Pulmonary Medicine. 2001;**7**:314-322

[4] Wahidi MM, Ravenel J, Palmer SM, McAdams HP. Progression of idiopathic pulmonary fibrosis in native lungs after single lung transplantation. Chest. 2002;**121**:2072-2076

[5] Toronto Lung Transplant G. Unilateral lung transplantation for pulmonary fibrosis. The New England Journal of Medicine. 1986;**314**:1140-1145

[6] Meyer DM, Edwards LB, Torres F, Jessen ME, Novick RJ. Impact of recipient age and procedure type on survival after lung transplantation for pulmonary fibrosis. The Annals of Thoracic Surgery. 2005;**79**:950-957 discussion 957-958

[7] Raghu G, Collard HR, Egan JJ, Martinez FJ, Behr J, Brown KK, et al. An official ATS/ERS/JRS/ALAT statement: Idiopathic pulmonary fibrosis: Evidence-based guidelines for diagnosis and management. American Journal of Respiratory and Critical Care Medicine. 2011;**183**:788-824

[8] Elicker BM, Golden JA, Ordovas KG, Leard L, Golden TR, Hays SR. Progression of native lung fibrosis in lung transplant recipients with idiopathic pulmonary fibrosis. Respiratory Medicine. 2010;**104**:426-433

[9] O'Beirne S, Counihan IP, Keane MP. Interstitial lung disease and lung transplantation. Seminars in Respiratory and Critical Care Medicine. 2010;**31**:139-146

[10] Hosenpud JD, Bennett LE, Keck BM, Fiol B, Boucek MM, Novick RJ. The registry of the International Society for Heart and Lung Transplantation: Sixteenth official report—1999. The Journal of Heart and Lung Transplantation. 1999;**18**:611-626

[11] Glanville AR, Estenne M. Indications, patient selection and timing of referral for lung transplantation. The European Respiratory Journal. 2003;**22**:845-852

[12] Rinaldi M, Sansone F, Boffini M, El Qarra S, Solidoro P, Cavallo N, et al. Single versus double lung transplantation in pulmonary fibrosis: A debated topic. Transplantation Proceedings. 2008;**40**:2010-2012

[13] Orens JB, Estenne M, Arcasoy S, Conte JV, Corris P, Egan JJ, et al. International Guidelines for the selection of lung transplant candidates: 2006 update—A consensus report from the Pulmonary Scientific Council of the International Society for Heart and Lung Transplantation. The Journal of Heart and Lung Transplantation. 2006;**25**:745-755

[14] Egan TM, Murray S, Bustami RT, Shearon TH, McCullough KP, Edwards LB, et al. Development of the new lung allocation system in the United States. American Journal of Transplantation. 2006;**6**:1212-1227

[15] Monaghan H, Wells AU, Colby TV, du Bois RM, Hansell DM, Nicholson AG. Prognostic implications of

histologic patterns in multiple surgical lung biopsies from patients with idiopathic interstitial pneumonias. Chest. 2004;**125**:522-526

[16] Mogulkoc N, Brutsche MH, Bishop PW, Greaves SM, Horrocks AW, Egan JJ, et al. Pulmonary function in idiopathic pulmonary fibrosis and referral for lung transplantation. American Journal of Respiratory and Critical Care Medicine. 2001;**164**:103-108

[17] Lama VN, Flaherty KR, Toews GB, Colby TV, Travis WD, Long Q , et al. Prognostic value of desaturation during a 6-minute walk test in idiopathic interstitial pneumonia. American Journal of Respiratory and Critical Care Medicine. 2003;**168**:1084-1090

[18] Flaherty KR, Travis WD, Colby TV, Toews GB, Kazerooni EA, Gross BH, et al. Histopathologic variability in usual and nonspecific interstitial pneumonias. American Journal of Respiratory and Critical Care Medicine. 2001;**164**:1722-1727

[19] Flaherty KR, Toews GB, Travis WD, Colby TV, Kazerooni EA, Gross BH, et al. Clinical significance of histological classification of idiopathic interstitial pneumonia. The European Respiratory Journal. 2002;**19**:275-283

[20] Hosenpud JD, Bennett LE, Keck BM, Edwards EB, Novick RJ. Effect of diagnosis on survival benefit of lung transplantation for end-stage lung disease. Lancet. 1998;**351**:24-27

[21] De Meester J, Smits JM, Persijn GG, Haverich A. Listing for lung transplantation: Life expectancy and transplant effect, stratified by type of end-stage lung disease, the Eurotransplant experience. The Journal of Heart and Lung Transplantation. 2001;**20**:518-524

[22] Thabut G, Mal H, Castier Y, Groussard O, Brugiere O, Marrash-Chahla R, et al. Survival benefit of lung transplantation for patients with idiopathic pulmonary fibrosis. The Journal of Thoracic and Cardiovascular Surgery. 2003;**126**:469-475

[23] Lederer DJ, Arcasoy SM, Wilt JS, D'Ovidio F, Sonett JR, Kawut SM. Six-minute-walk distance predicts waiting list survival in idiopathic pulmonary fibrosis. American Journal of Respiratory and Critical Care Medicine. 2006;**174**:659-664

[24] Shitrit D, Rusanov V, Peled N, Amital A, Fuks L, Kramer MR. The 15-step oximetry test: A reliable tool to identify candidates for lung transplantation among patients with idiopathic pulmonary fibrosis. The Journal of Heart and Lung Transplantation. 2009;**28**:328-333

[25] Eberlein M, Permutt S, Chahla MF, Bolukbas S, Nathan SD, Shlobin OA, et al. Lung size mismatch in bilateral lung transplantation is associated with allograft function and bronchiolitis obliterans syndrome. Chest. 2012;**141**:451-460

[26] Eberlein M, Reed RM, Permutt S, Chahla MF, Bolukbas S, Nathan SD, et al. Parameters of donor-recipient size mismatch and survival after bilateral lung transplantation. The Journal of Heart and Lung Transplantation. 2012;**31**:1207-1213, e1207

[27] Mason DP, Batizy LH, Wu J, Nowicki ER, Murthy SC, McNeill AM, et al. Matching donor to recipient in lung transplantation: How much does size matter? The Journal of Thoracic and Cardiovascular Surgery. 2009;**137**: 1234-1240 e1231

[28] Chaney J, Suzuki Y, Cantu E 3rd, van Berkel V. Lung donor selection criteria. Journal of Thoracic Disease. 2014;**6**:1032-1038

[29] Aguilar-Guisado M, Givalda J, Ussetti P, Ramos A, Morales P, Blanes M, et al. Pneumonia after lung

transplantation in the RESITRA Cohort: A multicenter prospective study. American Journal of Transplantation. 2007;7:1989-1996

[30] Remund KF, Best M, Egan JJ. Infections relevant to lung transplantation. Proceedings of the American Thoracic Society. 2009;6:94-100

[31] Mason DP, Rajeswaran J, Murthy SC, McNeill AM, Budev MM, Mehta AC, et al. Spirometry after transplantation: How much better are two lungs than one? The Annals of Thoracic Surgery. 2008;85:1193-1201, 1201 e1191-1192

[32] Fakhro M, Ingemansson R, Algotsson L, Lindstedt S. Impact of forced expiratory volume in 1 second (FEV1) and 6-minute walking distance at 3, 6, and 12 months and annually on survival and occurrence of bronchiolitis obliterans syndrome (BOS) after lung transplantation. Annals of Transplantation. 2017;22:532-540

[33] Becker FS, Martinez FJ, Brunsting LA, Deeb GM, Flint A, Lynch JP 3rd. Limitations of spirometry in detecting rejection after single-lung transplantation. American Journal of Respiratory and Critical Care Medicine. 1994;150:159-166

[34] Martinez JA, Paradis IL, Dauber JH, Grgurich W, Richards T, Yousem SA, et al. Spirometry values in stable lung transplant recipients. American Journal of Respiratory and Critical Care Medicine. 1997;155:285-290

[35] de Wall C, Sabine D, Gregor W, Mark G, Axel H, Thomas F, et al. Home spirometry as early detector of azithromycin refractory bronchiolitis obliterans syndrome in lung transplant recipients. Respiratory Medicine. 2014;108:405-412

[36] Robson KS, West AJ. Improving survival outcomes in lung transplant

recipients through early detection of bronchiolitis obliterans: Daily home spirometry versus standard pulmonary function testing. Canadian Journal of Respiratory Therapy. 2014;50:17-22

[37] Belloli EA, Wang X, Murray S, Forrester G, Weyhing A, Lin J, et al. Longitudinal forced vital capacity monitoring as a prognostic adjunct after lung transplantation. American Journal of Respiratory and Critical Care Medicine. 2015;192:209-218

[38] Chambers DC, Yusen RD, Cherikh WS, Goldfarb SB, Kucheryavaya AY, Khusch K, et al. The registry of the International Society for Heart and Lung Transplantation: Thirty-fourth adult lung and heart-lung transplantation Report-2017; focus theme: Allograft ischemic time. The Journal of Heart and Lung Transplantation. 2017;36:1047-1059

[39] Thabut G, Mal H. Outcomes after lung transplantation. Journal of Thoracic Disease. 2017;9:2684-2691

[40] Trulock EP, Edwards LB, Taylor DO, Boucek MM, Keck BM, Hertz MI. Registry of the International Society for Heart and Lung Transplantation: Twenty-second official adult lung and heart-lung transplant report—2005. The Journal of Heart and Lung Transplantation. 2005;24:956-967

[41] Yusen RD, Edwards LB, Kucheryavaya AY, Benden C, Dipchand AI, Goldfarb SB, et al. The registry of the International Society for Heart and Lung Transplantation: Thirty-second official adult lung and heart-lung transplantation report—2015; focus theme: Early graft failure. The Journal of Heart and Lung Transplantation. 2015;34:1264-1277

[42] Titman A, Rogers CA, Bonser RS, Banner NR, Sharples LD. Disease-specific survival benefit of lung transplantation in adults: A national

cohort study. American Journal of Transplantation. 2009;**9**:1640-1649

[43] Liu V, Zamora MR, Dhillon GS, Weill D. Increasing lung allocation scores predict worsened survival among lung transplant recipients. American Journal of Transplantation. 2010;**10**:915-920

[44] Edwards LB, Keck BM. Thoracic organ transplantation in the US. Clinical Transplants. 2002:29-40

[45] Chen H, Shiboski SC, Golden JA, Gould MK, Hays SR, Hoopes CW, et al. Impact of the lung allocation score on lung transplantation for pulmonary arterial hypertension. American Journal of Respiratory and Critical Care Medicine. 2009;**180**:468-474

[46] McCurry KR, Shearon TH, Edwards LB, Chan KM, Sweet SC, Valapour M, et al. Lung transplantation in the United States, 1998-2007. American Journal of Transplantation. 2009;**9**:942-958

[47] Thabut G, Christie JD, Ravaud P, Castier Y, Dauriat G, Jebrak G, et al. Survival after bilateral versus single-lung transplantation for idiopathic pulmonary fibrosis. Annals of Internal Medicine. 2009;**151**:767-774

[48] Freitas MC. Trend in lung transplantation in the U.S.: An analysis of the UNOS registry. Clinical Transplants. 2010:17-33

[49] Nathan SD, Barnett SD, Urban BA, Nowalk C, Moran BR, Burton N. Pulmonary embolism in idiopathic pulmonary fibrosis transplant recipients. Chest. 2003;**123**:1758-1763

[50] Schachna L, Medsger TAJ, Dauber JH, Wigley FM, Braunstein NA, White B, et al. Lung transplantation in scleroderma compared with idiopathic pulmonary fibrosis and idiopathic pulmonary arterial hypertension.

Arthritis and Rheumatism. 2006;**54**:3954-3961

[51] Burton CM, Carlsen J, Mortensen J, Andersen CB, Milman N, Iversen M. Long-term survival after lung transplantation depends on development and severity of bronchiolitis obliterans syndrome. The Journal of Heart and Lung Transplantation. 2007;**26**:681-686

[52] Di Giuseppe M, Gambelli F, Hoyle GW, Lungarella G, Studer SM, Richards T, et al. Systemic inhibition of NF-kappaB activation protects from silicosis. PLoS One. 2009;**4**:e5689

[53] Keating D, Levvey B, Kotsimbos T, Whitford H, Westall G, Williams T, et al. Lung transplantation in pulmonary fibrosis: Challenging early outcomes counterbalanced by surprisingly good outcomes beyond 15 years. Transplantation Proceedings. 2009;**41**:289-291

[54] Algar FJ, Espinosa D, Moreno P, Illana J, Cerezo F, Alvarez A, et al. Results of lung transplantation in idiopathic pulmonary fibrosis patients. Transplantation Proceedings. 2010;**42**:3211-3213

[55] Neurohr C, Huppmann P, Thum D, Leuschner W, von Wulffen W, Meis T, et al. Munich lung transplant G. potential functional and survival benefit of double over single lung transplantation for selected patients with idiopathic pulmonary fibrosis. Transplant International. 2010;**23**:887-896

[56] Machuca TN, Schio SM, Camargo SM, Lobato V, Costa CD, Felicetti JC, et al. Prognostic factors in lung transplantation: The Santa casa de Porto Alegre experience. Transplantation. 2011;**91**:1297-1303

[57] Nathan SD, Shlobin OA, Weir N, Ahmad S, Kaldjob JM, Battle E,

et al. Long-term course and prognosis of idiopathic pulmonary fibrosis in the new millennium. Chest. 2011;**140**:221-229

[58] Rivera-Lebron BN, Forfia PR, Kreider M, Lee JC, Holmes JH, Kawut SM. Echocardiographic and hemodynamic predictors of mortality in idiopathic pulmonary fibrosis. Chest. 2013;**144**:564-570

[59] Weiss ES, Allen JG, Merlo CA, Conte JV, Shah AS. Survival after single versus bilateral lung transplantation for high-risk patients with pulmonary fibrosis. The Annals of Thoracic Surgery. 2009;**88**:1616-1625 discussion 1625-1616

[60] Christie JD, Edwards LB, Kucheryavaya AY, Benden C, Dobbels F, Kirk R, et al. The registry of the International Society for Heart and Lung Transplantation: Twenty-eighth adult lung and heart-lung transplant report—2011. The Journal of Heart and Lung Transplantation. 2011;**30**:1104-1122

[61] Yusen RD, Edwards LB, Dipchand AI, Goldfarb SB, Kucheryavaya AY, Levvey BJ, et al. The registry of the International Society for Heart and Lung Transplantation: Thirty-third adult lung and heart-lung transplant Report-2016; focus theme: Primary diagnostic indications for transplant. The Journal of Heart and Lung Transplantation. 2016;**35**:1170-1184

[62] Christie JD, Edwards LB, Kucheryavaya AY, Benden C, Dipchand AI, Dobbels F, et al. The registry of the International Society for Heart and Lung Transplantation: 29th adult lung and heart-lung transplant report—2012. The Journal of Heart and Lung Transplantation. 2012;**31**:1073-1086

[63] Force SD, Kilgo P, Neujahr DC, Pelaez A, Pickens A, Fernandez FG, et al. Bilateral lung transplantation

offers better long-term survival, compared with single-lung transplantation, for younger patients with idiopathic pulmonary fibrosis. The Annals of Thoracic Surgery. 2011;**91**:244-249

[64] Weiss ES, Allen JG, Merlo CA, Conte JV, Shah AS. Factors indicative of long-term survival after lung transplantation: A review of 836 10-year survivors. The Journal of Heart and Lung Transplantation. 2010;**29**:240-246

[65] Mason DP, Brizzio ME, Alster JM, McNeill AM, Murthy SC, Budev MM, et al. Lung transplantation for idiopathic pulmonary fibrosis. The Annals of Thoracic Surgery. 2007;**84**:1121-1128

[66] Trulock EP, Edwards LB, Taylor DO, Boucek MM, Keck BM, Hertz MI, et al. Registry of the International Society for Heart and Lung Transplantation: Twenty-third official adult lung and heart-lung transplantation report—2006. The Journal of Heart and Lung Transplantation. 2006;**25**:880-892

[67] Nwakanma LU, Simpkins CE, Williams JA, Chang DC, Borja MC, Conte JV, et al. Impact of bilateral versus single lung transplantation on survival in recipients 60 years of age and older: Analysis of united network for organ sharing database. The Journal of Thoracic and Cardiovascular Surgery. 2007;**133**:541-547

[68] De Oliveira NC, Osaki S, Maloney J, Cornwell RD, Meyer KC. Lung transplant for interstitial lung disease: Outcomes before and after implementation of the united network for organ sharing lung allocation scoring system. European Journal of Cardio-Thoracic Surgery. 2012;**41**:680-685

[69] Smits JM, Vanhaecke J, Haverich A, de Vries E, Smith M, Rutgrink E, et al. Three-year survival rates for all consecutive heart-only and lung-only transplants performed in

Eurotransplant, 1997-1999. Clinical Transplants. 2003:89-100

[70] Date H, Tanimoto Y, Goto K, Yamadori I, Aoe M, Sano Y, et al. A new treatment strategy for advanced idiopathic interstitial pneumonia: Living-donor lobar lung transplantation. Chest. 2005;**128**:1364-1370

[71] Fakhro M, Ingemansson R, Skog I, Algotsson L, Hansson L, Koul B, Gustafsson R, Wierup P, Lindstedt S. 25-year follow-up after lung transplantation at Lund University Hospital in Sweden: Superior results obtained for patients with cystic fibrosis. Interact Cardiovasc Thorac Surg. Jul, 2016;**23**(1):65-73

[72] Wille KM, Gaggar A, Hajari AS, Leon KJ, Barney JB, Smith KH, et al. Bronchiolitis obliterans syndrome and survival following lung transplantation for patients with sarcoidosis. Sarcoidosis, Vasculitis, and Diffuse Lung Diseases. 2008;**25**:117-124

[73] Saggar R, Khanna D, Furst DE, Belperio JA, Park GS, Weigt SS, et al. Systemic sclerosis and bilateral lung transplantation: A single Centre experience. The European Respiratory Journal. 2010;**36**:893-900

[74] Grossman RF, Frost A, Zamel N, Patterson GA, Cooper JD, Myron PR, et al. Results of single-lung transplantation for bilateral pulmonary fibrosis. The Toronto Lung Transplant Group. The New England Journal of Medicine. 1990;**322**:727-733

[75] Vicente R, Morales P, Ramos F, Sole A, Mayo M, Villalain C. Perioperative complications of lung transplantation in patients with emphysema and fibrosis: Experience from 1992-2002. Transplantation Proceedings. 2006;**38**: 2560-2562

[76] de Perrot M, Chaparro C, McRae K, Waddell TK, Hadjiliadis D, Singer LG, et al. Twenty-year experience of lung transplantation at a single center: Influence of recipient diagnosis on long-term survival. The Journal of Thoracic and Cardiovascular Surgery. 2004;**127**:1493-1501

[77] Christie JD, Edwards LB, Aurora P, Dobbels F, Kirk R, Rahmel AO, et al. The registry of the International Society for Heart and Lung Transplantation: Twenty-sixth official adult lung and heart-lung transplantation Report—2009. The Journal of Heart and Lung Transplantation. 2009;**28**:1031-1049

[78] Lee JC, Christie JD. Primary graft dysfunction. Clinics in Chest Medicine. 2011;**32**:279-293

[79] Arcasoy SM, Fisher A, Hachem RR, Scavuzzo M, Ware LB, Dysfunction IWGoPLG. Report of the ISHLT working group on primary lung graft dysfunction part V: Predictors and outcomes. The Journal of Heart and Lung Transplantation. 2005;**24**:1483-1488

[80] Daud SA, Yusen RD, Meyers BF, Chakinala MM, Walter MJ, Aloush AA, et al. Impact of immediate primary lung allograft dysfunction on bronchiolitis obliterans syndrome. American Journal of Respiratory and Critical Care Medicine. 2007;**175**:507-513

[81] Fiser SM, Kron IL, McLendon Long S, Kaza AK, Kern JA, Tribble CG. Early intervention after severe oxygenation index elevation improves survival following lung transplantation. The Journal of Heart and Lung Transplantation. 2001;**20**:631-636

[82] Fakhro M, Broberg E, Algotsson L, Hansson L, Koul B, Gustafsson R, et al. Double lung, unlike single lung transplantation might provide a protective effect on mortality and bronchiolitis obliterans syndrome. Journal of Cardiothoracic Surgery. 2017;**12**:100

[83] Haider Y, Yonan N, Mogulkoc N, Carroll KB, Egan JJ. Bronchiolitis obliterans syndrome in single lung transplant recipients—Patients with emphysema versus patients with idiopathic pulmonary fibrosis. The Journal of Heart and Lung Transplantation. 2002;**21**:327-333

[84] Lama VN, Murray S, Lonigro RJ, Toews GB, Chang A, Lau C, et al. Course of FEV(1) after onset of bronchiolitis obliterans syndrome in lung transplant recipients. American Journal of Respiratory and Critical Care Medicine. 2007;**175**:1192-1198

Chapter 4

Lung Transplant for Interstitial Lung Diseases

Brandon Nokes, Eugene Golts and Kamyar Afshar

Abstract

Lung transplant is an important treatment modality for select cases of advanced interstitial lung disease. However, the pre- and postoperative management requires several unique considerations. The decision to transplant is based largely on clinical severity of illness and the lung allocation score. Transplant improves overall mortality across the interstitial lung diseases, though not all ILD subtypes experience equal benefit from lung transplant. Broadly speaking, there is no difference in benefit between single- and bilateral-lung transplants, though we will discuss some important clinical nuances to this decision as well. Lastly, there are a number of immunosuppression, coagulation, and malignancy risk considerations that must be carefully understood in caring for the lung transplant patient. This chapter will provide a general overview of the indications for lung transplant, risk stratification for lung transplant across the interstitial lung diseases, as well as general postoperative management details.

Keywords: interstitial lung diseases, usual interstitial pneumonia, lung transplant, lung allocation score, immunosuppression

1. Introduction

Lung transplantation is a therapeutic surgical option for selected patients with severe pulmonary disease who are refractory to medical therapy and continue to have progressive clinical deterioration [1]. As is discussed elsewhere in this book, the idiopathic interstitial pneumonias (IIPs) that require lung transplantation include idiopathic pulmonary fibrosis (IPF)/usual interstitial pneumonia (UIP), nonspecific interstitial pneumonia (NSIP), and acute interstitial pneumonia (AIP). The non-IIP ILD groups that are routinely evaluated for lung transplant include sarcoidosis, hypersensitivity pneumonitis (HP), rheumatologically associated UIP and NSIP, as well as lymphangioleiomyomatosis (LAM).

The general guidelines for lung transplantation consideration include (1) high (>50%) risk of death from lung disease within 2 years without transplant, (2) high (>80%) likelihood of surviving at least 90 days after lung transplantation, and (3) high (>80%) likelihood of 5-year posttransplant survival from a general medical perspective provided that there is adequate graft function [1]. Within the United States, between 1995 and 2015, ILDs accounted for 29.7% (n = 14,828) of lung transplants [1]. Collectively, the ILDs were the second most common indication for transplant behind chronic obstructive pulmonary disease without alpha-1-antitrypsin deficiency [1]. Of those patients, 6956 received single-lung transplant, and 7872 received bilateral-lung transplants [1]. Importantly, the ILD diagnostic subclasses were subdivided into idiopathic interstitial pneumonias (IIP) (n = 12,243) as well

Immunosuppressant Agent	Drug Interactions
Calcineurin Inhibitors: cyclosporin or tacrolimus	*Increased CNI levels:* allopurinol, azole antifungals, calcium channel blockers, colchicines, lansoprazole, macrolides, rabeprazole *Decreased CNI levels:* Barbiturates, carbamazepine, eiconacandins phenytoin, rifampin, rifabutin, St. John's wort, ticlopidine
Azathioprine	Allopurinol and ACE inhibitors slow azathioprine elimination thereby causing bone marrow suppression
Mycophenolate mofetil	Proton pump inhibitors reduce MPA peak concentrations. Norfloxacin & metronidazole combination reduce MPA trough concentrations. Rifampin reduces MPA exposure

Table 1.
Common drug-drug interactions with immunosuppressants—adapted from [37].

as ILD, not-IIP (n = 2585) (**Table 1**). Sarcoidosis, obliterative bronchiolitis (OB), and connective tissue disorder (CTD) were also listed diagnostic indications, and so there exists the potential for overlapping and misclassification of the underlying disease leading to lung transplant in a small proportion of cases. Irrespective of the subtype, ILDs present a unique challenge from pretransplant selection to postoperative care. The pre- and posttransplant clinical courses for each of these pathologies will be detailed within this chapter.

2. The lung allocation score (LAS) and the decision to transplant

An important part of the preoperative evaluation is individual assessment of patient risk with and without transplant. Some European countries, like France and Switzerland, have a national urgency list. Others, including the United Kingdom, allocate donor lungs according to individual transplant center decisions. More than 60% of the worldwide lung transplant activity, however, is allocated by the lung allocation score (LAS) [2]. The LAS has been adopted in many countries as a means of minimizing waitlist mortality [2]. The LAS is a calculated score (from 0 to 100) used to predict waitlist survival probability with and without a lung transplant for patients over the age of 12. Higher LAS scores impart a higher likelihood of waitlist mortality and allow for a prognostic stratification within regional transplant wait-lists and associated organ allocation preference [2]. This multifactorial system combines pulmonary function data with clinical comorbidity data. The implementation of this system has resulted in a substantial reduction in waitlist mortality and for the more expeditious mobilization of organs on a needs-based assessment [3]. Moreover, the median waitlist time in the United States has dropped from 4.1 to 2.1 months since the adoption of the LAS [2]. As such, the LAS has since been adopted in a number of other countries' transplant programs [4, 5]. Similar OLT outcomes research has been conducted on healthcare-related quality of life (HRQL) after transplant, and in general, higher LAS imparts a greater improvement in HRQL after OLT [6]. This benefit appears to diminish with greater age, especially after age 65 [6].

Despite the shorter waitlist time with higher LAS score, some patients may remain on the waitlist for longer periods of time. This is a reflection of a number of logistic limitations underpinning the lung transplant process. Notably, the number of available lung allografts does not meet the current US or global need. Up to

20% of lung transplant candidates are inactivated or die before an adequate donor becomes available [7]. Moreover, explanted lungs are inherently fragile, which further complicates the transplant process. Recipient underlying lung disease greatly matters in the type of transplant procedure required, e.g., unilateral vs. bilateral OLT. Donor and recipient lung size match is essential for adequate function of the allograft as well as survival [8]. Shorter patients may require lung donors from pediatric patients. However, pediatric lungs are first offered to pediatric candidates (age < 18 years) before they become available to other potential recipients.

Donors and recipient ABO blood type and human leukocyte antigen (HLA) compatibility must also be considered. Ideally, patients will have absent panel-reactive antibodies (PRA). Notably, only 69.8% of lung transplant candidates had 0% PRA since 2009. Patients with a higher PRA, particularly PRA greater than 25%, have a higher 30-day and overall mortality [9]. This makes the waitlist time for an appropriate crossmatch significantly longer and can potentially exclude the candidate from transplantation due to elevated risk of rejection.

The underlying diagnosis necessitating transplant also impacts the LAS. With respect to ILD, individuals with IPF and sarcoidosis are more likely to have a higher LAS than more common diagnoses such as COPD [3]. With LAS scores greater than 60, individuals with IPF have a greater risk of posttransplant mortality. Although no strict stratification exists to say at which LAS transplant should be avoided, this decision is left to local transplant centers when the risk is exceedingly high [3].

3. Idiopathic pulmonary fibrosis (IPF) lung transplant overview

Given the relative preponderance of IPF as a pretransplant diagnosis in comparison to the other ILDs, a brief overview of IPF outcomes following transplant is included here. The most common of the ILDs to necessitate transplant is IPF, which accounts for roughly 46% of patients on the lung transplant waiting list according to 2011 data from the Organ Procurement and Transplantation Network (OPTN) [10]. Importantly, IPF has no definitive treatment and an average survival of 2–3 years after diagnosis. It is associated with older age, male sex, and smoking history. It has also been associated with shortened telomere length, both in familial and sporadic forms [11]. This finding has been demonstrated in both peripheral blood leukocytes and postmortem lung tissue samples [11]. There are no targeted therapies readily available to curtail this epigenetic proclivity, but as IPF progresses, OLT remains a life-saving measure, with a median survival of 4.5 years after transplant for both bilateral- (BLT) and single-lung transplant (SLT) [12]. A recent meta-analysis suggested that those with BLT may have improved survival when compared to SLT, but this may be a result of selection bias [12]. Importantly, only those with end-stage bronchiectasis and idiopathic pulmonary arterial hypertension (IPAH) require BLT, and essentially all other diagnoses are suitable for SLT [12].

The clinical time course for IPF is heterogeneous, but there is invariably a clinical and functional decline, and many of these patients will have to go for transplant (**Figure 1**) [13]. The survival after transplant is the poorest for IPF relative to other indications for OLT, with the exception of re-transplant (**Figure 2**) [1]. As noted, the implementation of the LAS has allowed more rapid allocation of allografts for IPF and has improved prognosis tremendously. Further, although the median FVC for IPF at time of transplant is ~40–45%, this improves to 65% after transplant, contingent on selecting appropriate donor size [14]. Predicted total lung capacity (pTLC) can be used to approximate appropriate donor lung size for SLT or BLT [14]. In the absence of postoperative graft dysfunction, improvements can also be expected in HRQL, 6-minute walk test (6MWT), PaO2, and dyspnea severity [15, 16].

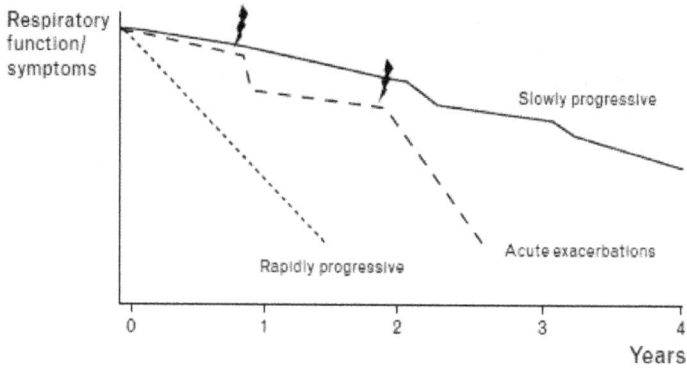

Figure 1.
Clinical course of patients with idiopathic pulmonary fibrosis. Many follow the course of the slow progressive decline. A minority will have a rapidly progressive course. An acute exacerbation can occur at any point in the course of functional decline. Rapidly progressive; acute exacerbations; and slowly progressive. Adapted from [51].

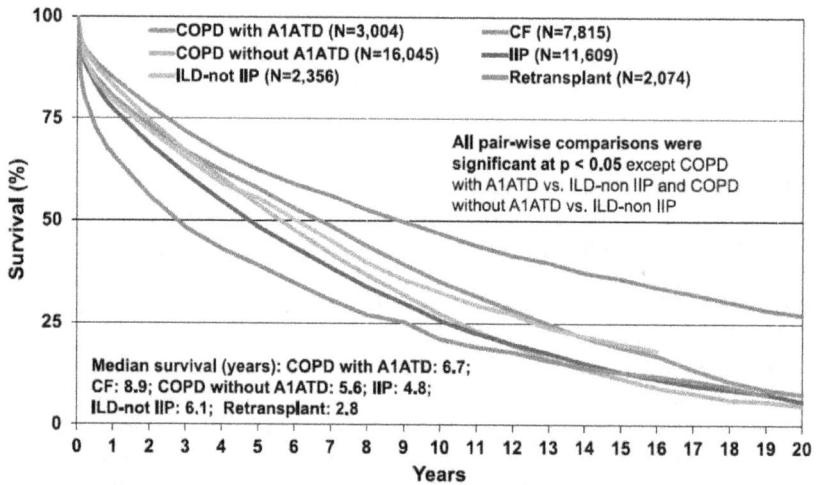

Figure 2.
Kaplan-Meier survival by diagnosis for adult lung transplants performed between January 1990 and June 2010. Alpha-1, α1-antitrypsin deficiency emphysema; CF, cystic fibrosis; COPD, chronic obstructive pulmonary disease; IPF, idiopathic pulmonary fibrosis; PAH, pulmonary arterial hypertension—adapted from [38].

4. Issues addressed while awaiting lung transplantation

4.1 Short telomere length

Rare mutations in the telomere pathways (NAD1, PARN, RTELI, TERC, TERT) are found in familial pulmonary fibrosis [11, 17]. Having short telomere length is characterized by earlier onset of IPF, associated liver disease, impaired CMV immunity, and bone marrow suppression [11, 17, 18]. Newton et al. conducted an observation cohort study of IPF patients who underwent lung transplantation [19]. Patients were stratified into two groups based on the telomere length; 32 patients were in Group 1 (telomere length < 10th percentile). They were compared to the 56 patients in Group 2 (telomere length ≥ 10th percentile). There were no difference between the two groups with regard to baseline demographics and severity of lung disease.

Group 1 lung transplant recipients had higher incidence of primary graft dysfunction grade 3 and earlier time to chronic allograft dysfunction. There was no difference in the incidence of acute allograft rejection, cytopenias, or infections. Popescu et al. reported the increased risk of *Cytomegalovirus* (CMV) infections in the short telomere IPF lung transplant recipients [18]. Given this knowledge, some lung transplant centers will only accept CMV-negative donor lungs in order to reduce risk of transmission and CMV-related complications. In the case series of eight patients by Silhan et al., these lung transplant recipients with short telomere tolerated a dual drug immunosuppression [20]. The antimetabolites could be easily withdrawn. Hematological complications occurred in four lung transplant recipients, with two cases of known bone marrow failure prior to lung transplantation. There was a 12% platelet transfusion rate. Several patients had infectious complications with gram-negative pneumonia/sepsis, fungal infections, and CMV disease (pneumonitis). These patients developed acute kidney injury, with half of them requiring renal replacement therapy.

5. Studies on OFEV/Esbriet prior to lung transplantation

Many centers were initially reluctant to the use of nintedanib in IPF patient listed for lung transplant due to its potential to increase perioperative bleeding risk and impaired wound healing, thereby causing bronchial anastomotic complications. These concerns have been alleviated with recent publications that indicate no worsening of airway complications or bleeding risks [21, 22]. Four of the nine patients in Balestro et al.'s study required intraoperative venoarterial or veno-veno extracorporeal membrane oxygenation (ECMO) [21]. No patient experienced major bleeding, despite being on nintedanib as well as aspirin + clopidogrel. There were also no reports of airway anastomotic dehiscence.

The exact mechanism of action of pirfenidone may be from the inhibition of transforming growth factor beta (TGF-b) [23]. A few case reports describe the safety of pirfenidone use as a bridge to lung transplantation [24, 25].

Mortensen et al. reported the largest retrospective analysis of 18 IPF patients who took pirfenidone prior to lung transplantation [25]. Only one patient developed sternal dehiscence that was more related to a surgical issue. There was no airway dehiscence in any of the 18 patients.

6. Other preoperative immunosuppressive considerations

Many patients with sarcoidosis, hypersensitivity pneumonitis, and rheumatologically induced ILD require corticosteroids to help control respiratory symptoms and further lung parenchymal inflammation. Chronic steroid use can lead to thinning of the skin, myopathy, and delayed wound healing [26]. McAnally et al. reported the deleterious effects of pretransplant corticosteroids [27]. Sixty six percent of their patients awaiting lung transplantation were on corticosteroids. The 132 patients in the low-dose steroid group (<0.42 mg/kg/m^2) were compared to the 69 high-dose steroid group (≥0.42 mg/kg/m^2). Patients were clinically similar based on underlying lung disease, severity of lung function, transplant type, and donor lung ischemic time. The high-dose steroid group had higher rates of serious infections and delayed wound healing as well as higher risk of early posttransplant death. The general recommendations are not only to minimize the steroid dose to allow for continued stabilization of underlying ILD but also to minimize complications with bridge to lung transplantation.

Lymphangioleiomyomatosis is characterized by proliferation of LAM cells, the abnormal smooth muscle-like cells that metastasize to lead cystic changes seen on chest radiograph. The cysts are present throughout both lung fields, although they predominate in the lower lung region. Their size can vary from 3 mm up to 3 cm. Larger cysts (>0.5 cm) are more likely to cause pneumothoraces [28]. Pneumothoraces occur in up to 60–70% of women with LAM. A majority of first-time pneumothoraces occur in the third and fourth decade of life [29]. Unfortunately, they are not a one-time event for most LAM patients. Four percent of these individuals can have simultaneous bilateral pneumothoraces. Recurrence rates for pneumothoraces are upward of 70%. Sirolimus, an mTOR inhibitor, is currently recommended as therapy for LAM. It blocks the signaling pathway for the growth and proliferation of the LAM cells that cause all the clinical manifestations described. Common adverse events when taking sirolimus include mucositis, diarrhea, nausea, hypercholesterolemia, and lower extremity edema. The most relevant adverse events of sirolimus in the context of this chapter are poor wound healing and anastomotic dehiscence in perioperative periods [30–32]. Dilling et al. reported their experience of continued use of sirolimus in patients with LAM while awaiting lung transplantation [33]. All patients were continued on their maintenance sirolimus dose up to the day of lung transplantation. None of the patients developed increased bleeding or wound dehiscence. In select patients, the use of sirolimus may be required. Lymphangioleiomyomatosis can recur following lung transplantation. It may present itself primarily as a chylous effusion. If a single-lung transplant is performed, the cystic lung disease can continue to progress. Sirolimus can be added to the maintenance immunosuppression to help the underlying process. There is varying reports on the safety of sirolimus use in early post-lung transplantation [31, 34].

7. Medical care of the lung transplant patient

The medical care after OLT requires close coordination between a multidisciplinary transplant team, including but not limited to transplant pulmonologists, cardiothoracic surgeons, pharmacists, physical/occupational/respiratory therapists, social workers, transplant nurses, and patient advocates. The transplant committee decision-making process for transplant eligibility is complex and beyond the scope of this text. However, important consideration elements of note are functional status, including physical ability to tolerate and recover from OLT [1]. To this end, physical therapy and nutritional optimization are paramount in the pretransplant process in order to ensure posttransplant success. Many inpatients that are listed for transplant have achieved benefit from early veno-venous extracorporeal membranous oxygenation (VV-ECMO) in order to facilitate mobilization and engagement with physical therapy [35, 36].

Transplant infectious disease specialists can be helpful in directing regionally appropriate infectious disease screening/treatment prior to transplant. *Cytomegalovirus* (CMV) and Epstein-Barr virus (EBV) status assessments between donor and recipient are paramount in guiding postoperative antiviral therapy, with CMV +/− and CMV −/+ being prophylaxed with valganciclovir and CMV −/− receiving acyclovir. EBV status is helpful in determining immunosuppressive needs. Over-immunosuppression can increase the risk of posttransplant lymphoproliferative disorder (PTLD), a lymphoma-like condition that responds to reduction in immunosuppression. All lung transplant recipients receive high-dose glucocorticoid treatment and require pneumocystis prophylaxis, typically with trimethoprim-sulfamethoxazole.

7.1 Complications following lung transplant

Acute rejection rates are extremely common in the first year after lung transplantation with approximately 30–40% of recipients having at least one episode in the first year after transplant. Triple-drug immunosuppressive agents have become the standard of care and are prescribed to minimize this risk [37]. Immunosuppressive dosing must be carefully considered so as to minimize acute rejection risk without leading way to infections. The regimen typically prescribed in lung and most solid organ transplants typically includes prednisone, a calcineurin inhibitor (tacrolimus or cyclosporine), and an antimetabolite (azathioprine or mycophenolate mofetil). Despite the unique side effects of each of these drug classes, the cumulative effect of immunosuppression may predispose individuals to opportunistic infections, renal failure, malignancies, posttransplant hypertension, diabetes, and dyslipidemia. **Table 1** reviews common drug interactions that can alter immunosuppressant clearance or therapeutic drug levels.

The lung allograft is subject to a variety of insults resulting in various parenchymal abnormalities. These complications are broadly classified as infectious and noninfectious. The development of infections is the leading cause of morbidity and mortality in the first 3 years following lung transplantation [38]. Bacterial pathogens are the most common, but fungal and viral infections are also particularly important (especially *Aspergillus* and *Cytomegalovirus*).

Despite their ubiquitous and potentially ominous nature, radiographic pulmonary parenchymal abnormalities predicting posttransplant complication can be nonspecific (**Figures 3–5**). Bacterial and fungal radiographic features are highly varied and include consolidation, ill-defined nodules, cavitation, and ground-glass opacifications, making them difficult to identify. Viral infections (especially CMV) may have normal radiographs. They can also show ground-glass, micronodules, consolidation, and/or reticulonodular opacities.

Moreover, acute cellular rejection (ACR) can present similar to any of the previously mentioned complications. ACR radiographic features can appear as normal radiograph, ground-glass opacities, alveolar opacities, consolidation, nodules, as well as a new or evolving pleural effusion (seen in 43% of patients) [39, 40].

Due to the radiographic overlap in postoperative lung pathologies, broad-spectrum antimicrobial therapy is often instituted in the acutely ill lung transplant

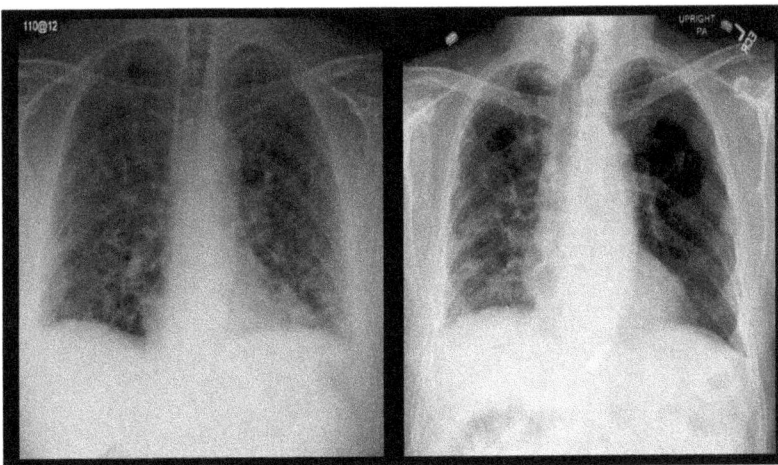

Figure 3.
Chest X-ray of a single-lung transplant recipient for IPF.

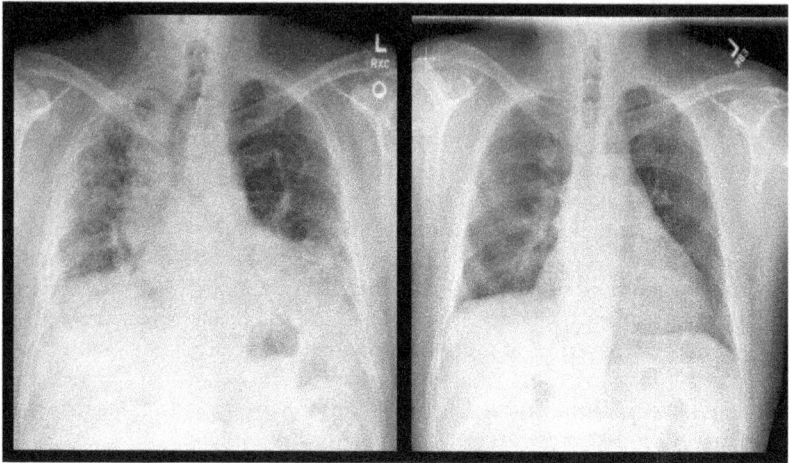

Figure 4.
Chest X-ray of a bilateral-lung transplant recipient for IPF.

recipient. A broad infectious differential must be maintained given the triple-drug immunosuppression when considering treatment options. Similarly, acute rejection is on the differential, and differentiating between the two is imperative. Clinical correlation and transbronchial biopsy are often indicated for discerning the diagnosis. The number of acute cellular rejections and infections contribute to a higher risk of developing chronic rejection.

Primary graft dysfunction (PGD) accounts for the main cause of death within the first 30 days following lung transplantation [38]. The underlying diagnosis leading to transplant is not predictive of developing PGD (restrictive disease with PGD 22.1% vs. without PGD 20.3%) [37]. More recently, patients with IPF and associated pulmonary hypertension have been shown to have a higher incidence of developing PGD [41]. Moreover, higher pulmonary artery pressures impart a greater risk of developing severe PGD (grade 3).

Early diagnosis and management may impart a lower incidence of chronic allograft rejection. Chronic allograft rejection manifests as bronchiolitis

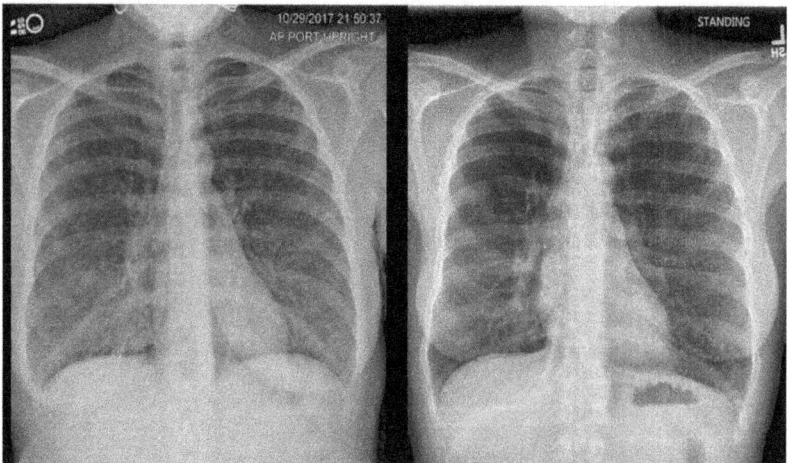

Figure 5.
Chest X-ray of a single right-lung transplant recipient for LAM.

obliterans syndrome (BOS) or restrictive allograft syndrome (RAS). BOS is typically a progressive airflow limitation demonstrated on pulmonary function testing (PFT). Grading of BOS depends on the severity of airflow limitation relative to the patient's best posttransplant FEV_1. The radiographic presentations of BOS include a mixture of hypo- and hyperattenuation (mosaic attenuation) regions produced by air trapping and decreased peripheral vascularity, bronchiectasis, and subsegmental atelectasis. RAS is hallmarked by upper lobe fibrosis. Radiographic RAS may have reticulonodular opacities, honeycombing, traction bronchiectasis, loss of lung volume, and interlobular septal thickening (**Figure 6**). In comparison to BOS however, these patients have restrictive physiology on PFTs [40, 42].

By bronchoscopy, the presence of eosinophilia and neutrophilia, airway infection and/or colonization, and acute cellular/lymphocytic bronchiolitis all impart increased risk of developing both BOS and RAS [37]. The underlying pathology necessitating transplant does not seem to influence the development of one form of chronic allograft rejection (24% BOS and 20.8% RAS).

Altering medications within therapeutic classes or augmenting existing therapy has been advocated when patients develop chronic rejection. There is clearly a small subset of patients who derive benefit from this therapy. However, alteration of immunosuppression may also increase the risk of opportunistic infections and development malignancy.

One alternative therapy for BOS is chronic azithromycin. Several small case series as well as one prospective, randomized, double-blind, placebo-controlled trial have suggested a benefit with azithromycin in lung transplant recipients [43–45]. Azithromycin may prevent the development of BOS, as well as treat a subset of patients with BOS. The mechanism for the positive effect of azithromycin in BOS prevention and treatment is believed to be related to its anti-inflammatory properties. Chronic azithromycin therapy is well tolerated. Gastrointestinal side effects, QTc prolongation, and auditory disturbances are common side effects. Clinicians should be aware that this medication is often taken chronically in lung transplant patients when considering antibiotic choices for acute respiratory infections in this population.

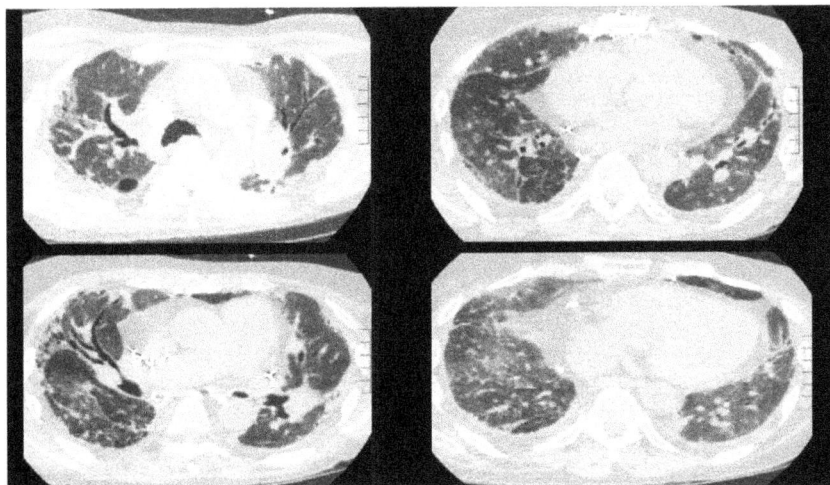

Figure 6.
CT chest for a bilateral-lung transplant recipient for sarcoidosis in chronic allograft rejection.

7.2 Airway complications

Currently, the bronchial anastomosis is created in an "end-to-end" fashion, and bronchial artery circulation is lost. Thus, the donor bronchus and anastomosis depend solely on the poorly oxygenated pulmonary artery, portending to the development of local ischemia. Early complications (<3 months) from airway/anastomotic ischemia include necrosis and wound dehiscence. During the healing and remodeling phase (>3 months), typical complications are airway stenosis, granulation tissue accumulation, and malacia (typically a later occurrence). Graft rejection, immunosuppression, and bronchopulmonary infections have also been associated with airway complications. Lung transplant-associated airway complications manifest in up to 30% of patients [46, 47]. Management strategies include airway dilation with silicone or self-expandable metallic stents, cryoablation, and laser photoresection. Airway stents are generally placed when respiratory symptoms are refractory to the abovementioned modalities (**Figure 7**). Most patients experience improvement in symptoms and lung function. However, complications from the above interventions include mucus plugging, obstructive granuloma, stent migration, fracture, or infectious colonization.

7.3 Complications of native lung in single-lung transplantation

It bears mention that patients' native lung disease progression is not halted with the contralateral lung transplantation despite robust immunosuppression. The amount of native lung ground-glass opacification or fibrosis does not change or increases for the majority of single-lung transplant recipients with IPF [48]. Patients with IPF lose 10.8% of native lung volume and have an 11% increase in fibrosis in the first 4 years following SLT [49]. Up to 52% of the native lungs had evidence of fibrosis at the time of transplant, and this number grows to 92% at 4 years posttransplant.

Common complications reported in IPF patients following SLT include bacterial or fungal infections, retention of secretions with associated airway obstruction and atelectasis, as well as pneumothoraces [50]. Moreover, posttransplant acute exacerbation of IPF is increasingly recognized [51]. Bronchogenic carcinomas have been reported at higher rates in single-lung transplant recipients. Significant

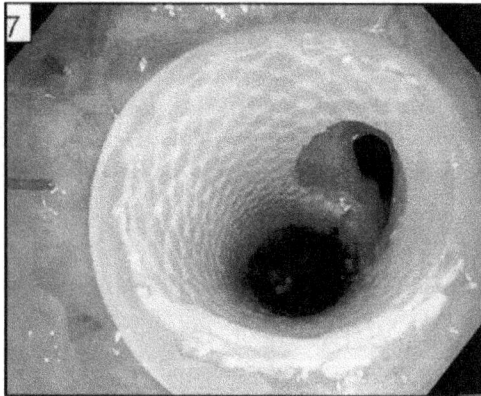

Figure 7.
Silicone endobronchial stent placed in a patient with anastomotic stricture development.

contributing risk factors include advanced recipient or donor age, smoking history (>60 pack years), and COPD or IPF as the underlying lung disease [52].

7.4 Thromboembolic events following lung transplantation

Deep vein thrombus (DVT) and pulmonary emboli (PE) occur in up to 29% of lung transplant recipients. Two-thirds of these events occur in the first year of transplantation, and 20% of these events develop within the first month. Reduced mobility and recent surgery are risk factors. Inflammation also inhibits anticoagulant factors [53]. Other risk factors include, most notably, an underlying diagnosis of IPF. Male gender, advanced age, pneumonia, diabetes mellitus, and utilization of cardiopulmonary bypass are other well-defined risk factors [41, 54]. Most of the pulmonary emboli occur within the allograft (86%) [54, 55].

The intrinsically thrombogenic surface of the allograft vasculature anastomosis and increased allograft perfusion with concurrent drop in pulmonary vascular resistance in single-lung transplant recipients are postulated predilections for allograft predominant clot formation. Notably, clots can still occur in the native lung. Most posttransplant PEs are 5.8 months following lung transplantation. Many centers advocate prophylactic anticoagulation for 6–9 months following transplant for this reason. Luckily, most patients tolerate an embolic event, even in the presence of large clot burden, without a loss of lung allograft function [56].

8. Conclusion

Lung transplantation is an important treatment option for patients with interstitial lung disease after medical therapy has failed. However, pulmonary fibrosis patients have the worst survival following lung transplantation. Nonetheless, there is a survival advantage for those with pulmonary fibrosis who proceed with lung transplant [57, 58]. Moreover, lung transplantation improves quality of life. ISHLT registry data denotes that lung transplant recipients have better quality of life, general health, and many are even able return to work. Up to 30% of patients are working at 1 year, and 50% are working at 5 years [59–62].

Lung transplantation, however, is not without its risks, and patient awareness of these risks is important before lung transplantation is entertained or pursued. All appropriate measures should be taken to mitigate risk factors surrounding lung transplantation. So doing can potentially improve long-term outcomes. Lastly, as a growing number of lung transplant recipients make their way into the community, the onus for and access to working lung transplant knowledge now extend far beyond the transplant center, into our communities at large.

Acknowledgements

Thank you to Sara Carey for your innumerable editorial contributions.

Conflict of interest

The authors have no conflicts of interest to disclose.

Author details

Brandon Nokes[1], Eugene Golts[2] and Kamyar Afshar[1*]

1 Division of Pulmonary, Critical Care, and Sleep Medicine, University of California San Diego, San Diego, CA, USA

2 Division of Cardiothoracic Surgery, University of California San Diego, San Diego, CA, USA

*Address all correspondence to: kaafshar@ucsd.edu

IntechOpen

References

[1] Yusen RD, Edwards LB, Dipchand AI, et al. The registry of the international society for heart and lung transplantation: Thirty-third adult lung and heart-lung transplant report-2016; Focus theme: Primary diagnostic indications for transplant. The Journal of Heart and Lung Transplantation. 2016;**35**:1170-1184

[2] Egan TM, Murray S, Bustami RT, et al. Development of the new lung allocation system in the United States. American Journal of Transplantation. 2006;**6**:1212-1227

[3] Liu V, Zamora MR, Dhillon GS, Weill D. Increasing lung allocation scores predict worsened survival among lung transplant recipients. American Journal of Transplantation. 2010;**10**:915-920

[4] Schuba B, Scheklinski M, von Dossow V, et al. Five-year experience using the lung allocation score: The Munich lung transplant group. European Journal of Cardio-Thoracic Surgery. 2018;**54**:328-333

[5] Gottlieb J, Smits J, Schramm R, et al. Lung transplantation in Germany since the introduction of the lung allocation score. Deutsches Ärzteblatt International. 2017;**114**:179-185

[6] Singer JP, Katz PP, Soong A, et al. Effect of lung transplantation on health-related quality of life in the era of the lung allocation score: A U.S. prospective cohort study. American Journal of Transplantation. 2017;**17**:1334-1345

[7] Sundaresan S, Trachiotis GD, Aoe M, Patterson GA, Cooper JD. Donor lung procurement: Assessment and operative technique. The Annals of Thoracic Surgery. 1993;**56**:1409-1413

[8] Eberlein M, Reed RM, Permutt S, et al. Parameters of donor-recipient size mismatch and survival after bilateral lung transplantation. The Journal of Heart and Lung Transplantation. 2012;**31**:1207-13.e7

[9] Shah AS, Nwakanma L, Simpkins C, Williams J, Chang DC, Conte JV. Pretransplant panel reactive antibodies in human lung transplantation: An analysis of over 10,000 patients. The Annals of Thoracic Surgery. 2008;**85**:1919-1924

[10] http://optn.transplant.hrsa.gov

[11] Snetselaar R, van Moorsel CHM, Kazemier KM, et al. Telomere length in interstitial lung diseases. Chest. 2015;**148**:1011-1018

[12] Kistler KD, Nalysnyk L, Rotella P, Esser D. Lung transplantation in idiopathic pulmonary fibrosis: A systematic review of the literature. BMC Pulmonary Medicine. 2014;**14**:139

[13] Afshar K, Sharma OP. Interstitial lung disease: Trials and tribulations. Current Opinion in Pulmonary Medicine. 2008;**14**:427-433

[14] Miyoshi S, Schaefers HJ, Trulock EP, et al. Donor selection for single and double lung transplantation. Chest size matching and other factors influencing posttransplantation vital capacity. Chest. 1990;**98**:308-313

[15] Thabut G, Mal H, Castier Y, et al. Survival benefit of lung transplantation for patients with idiopathic pulmonary fibrosis. The Journal of Thoracic and Cardiovascular Surgery. 2003;**126**:469-475

[16] Neurohr C, Huppmann P, Thum D, et al. Potential functional and survival benefit of double over single lung transplantation for selected patients with idiopathic pulmonary fibrosis. Transplant International. 2010;**23**:887-896

[17] Snetselaar R, van Batenburg AA, van Oosterhout MFM, et al. Short telomere length in IPF lung associates with fibrotic lesions and predicts survival. PLoS One. 2017;**12**:e0189467

[18] Popescu I, Mannem H, Winters SA, et al. Impaired CMV immunity in idiopathic pulmonary fibrosis lung transplant recipients with short telomeres. American Journal of Respiratory and Critical Care Medicine. 2018. https://www.ncbi.nlm.nih.gov/pubmed/30088779. [Epub ahead of print]

[19] Newton CA, Kozlitina J, Lines JR, Kaza V, Torres F, Garcia CK. Telomere length in patients with pulmonary fibrosis associated with chronic lung allograft dysfunction and post-lung transplantation survival. The Journal of Heart and Lung Transplantation. 2017;**36**:845-853

[20] Silhan LL, Shah PD, Chambers DC, et al. Lung transplantation in telomerase mutation carriers with pulmonary fibrosis. The European Respiratory Journal. 2014;**44**:178-187

[21] Balestro E, Solidoro P, Parigi P, Boffini M, Lucianetti A, Rea F. Safety of nintedanib before lung transplant: An Italian case series. Respirology Case Reports. 2018;**6**:e00312

[22] Lambers C, Boehm PM, Lee S, et al. Effect of antifibrotics on short-term outcome after bilateral lung transplantation: A multicentre analysis. The European Respiratory Journal. 21 Jun 2018;**51**(6). https://www.ncbi.nlm.nih.gov/pubmed/?term=lambers+effect+of+antifibrotics

[23] Takeda Y, Tsujino K, Kijima T, Kumanogoh A. Efficacy and safety of pirfenidone for idiopathic pulmonary fibrosis. Patient Preference and Adherence. 2014;**8**:361-370

[24] Paone G, Sebastiani A, Ialleni E, et al. A combined therapeutic approach in progressive idiopathic pulmonary fibrosis-pirfenidone as bridge therapy for ex vivo lung transplantation: A case report. Transplantation Proceedings. 2015;**47**:855-857

[25] Mortensen A, Cherrier L, Walia R. Effect of pirfenidone on wound healing in lung transplant patients. Multidisciplinary Respiratory Medicine. 2018;**13**:16

[26] Wang AS, Armstrong EJ, Armstrong AW. Corticosteroids and wound healing: Clinical considerations in the perioperative period. American Journal of Surgery. 2013;**206**:410-417

[27] McAnally KJ, Valentine VG, LaPlace SG, McFadden PM, Seoane L, Taylor DE. Effect of pre-transplantation prednisone on survival after lung transplantation. The Journal of Heart and Lung Transplantation. 2006;**25**:67-74

[28] Steagall WK, Glasgow CG, Hathaway OM, et al. Genetic and morphologic determinants of pneumothorax in lymphangioleiomyomatosis. American Journal of Physiology. Lung Cellular and Molecular Physiology. 2007;**293**:L800-L808

[29] Almoosa KF, Ryu JH, Mendez J, et al. Management of pneumothorax in lymphangioleiomyomatosis: Effects on recurrence and lung transplantation complications. Chest. 2006;**129**:1274-1281

[30] King-Biggs MB, Dunitz JM, Park SJ, Kay Savik S, Hertz MI. Airway anastomotic dehiscence associated with use of sirolimus immediately after lung transplantation. Transplantation. 2003;**75**:1437-1443

[31] Groetzner J, Kur F, Spelsberg F, et al. Airway anastomosis complications in de novo lung transplantation with sirolimus-based immunosuppression. The Journal of Heart and Lung Transplantation. 2004;**23**:632-638

[32] McCormack FX, Inoue Y, Moss J, et al. Efficacy and safety of sirolimus in lymphangioleiomyomatosis. The New England Journal of Medicine. 2011;**364**:1595-1606

[33] Dilling DF, Gilbert ER, Picken MM, Eby JM, Love RB, Le Poole IC. A current viewpoint of lymphangioleiomyomatosis supporting immunotherapeutic treatment options. American Journal of Respiratory Cell and Molecular Biology. 2012;**46**:1-5

[34] Wojarski J, Zeglen S, Ochman M, Karolak W. Early sirolimus-based immunosuppression is safe for lung transplantation patients: Retrospective, single arm, exploratory study. Annals of Transplantation. 2018;**23**:598-607

[35] Wickerson L, Rozenberg D, Janaudis-Ferreira T, et al. Physical rehabilitation for lung transplant candidates and recipients: An evidence-informed clinical approach. World Journal of Transplantation. 2016;**6**:517-531

[36] Wickerson L, Mathur S, Helm D, Singer L, Brooks D. Physical activity profile of lung transplant candidates with interstitial lung disease. Journal of Cardiopulmonary Rehabilitation and Prevention. 2013;**33**:106-112

[37] Afshar KON, Whelan T. Medical complications in lung transplant recipients with pulmonary fibrosis. Journal of Pulmonary & Respiratory Medicine. 2013;**3**:2. DOI: 10.4172/2161-105X.1000145. https://www.omicsonline.org/medical-complications-in-lung-transplant-recipients-with-pulmonary-fibrosis-2161-105X.1000145.pdf

[38] Goldfarb SB, Levvey BJ, Edwards LB, et al. The registry of the international society for heart and lung transplantation: Nineteenth pediatric lung and heart-lung transplantation report-2016; Focus theme: Primary diagnostic indications for transplant.

The Journal of Heart and Lung Transplantation. 2016;**35**:1196-1205

[39] Loubeyre P, Revel D, Delignette A, Loire R, Mornex JF. High-resolution computed tomographic findings associated with histologically diagnosed acute lung rejection in heart-lung transplant recipients. Chest. 1995;**107**:132-138

[40] Krishnam MS, Suh RD, Tomasian A, et al. Postoperative complications of lung transplantation: Radiologic findings along a time continuum. Radiographics. 2007;**27**:957-974

[41] Fang A, Studer S, Kawut SM, et al. Elevated pulmonary artery pressure is a risk factor for primary graft dysfunction following lung transplantation for idiopathic pulmonary fibrosis. Chest. 2011;**139**:782-787

[42] Pakhale SS, Hadjiliadis D, Howell DN, et al. Upper lobe fibrosis: A novel manifestation of chronic allograft dysfunction in lung transplantation. The Journal of Heart and Lung Transplantation. 2005;**24**:1260-1268

[43] Gerhardt SG, McDyer JF, Girgis RE, Conte JV, Yang SC, Orens JB. Maintenance azithromycin therapy for bronchiolitis obliterans syndrome: Results of a pilot study. American Journal of Respiratory and Critical Care Medicine. 2003;**168**:121-125

[44] Kanazawa S, Nomura S, Muramatsu M, Yamaguchi K, Fukuhara S. Azithromycin and bronchiolitis obliterans. American Journal of Respiratory and Critical Care Medicine. 2004;**169**:654-655. Author reply 5

[45] Verleden GM, Dupont LJ. Azithromycin therapy for patients with bronchiolitis obliterans syndrome after lung transplantation. Transplantation. 2004;**77**:1465-1467

[46] Santacruz JF, Mehta AC. Airway complications and management

after lung transplantation: Ischemia, dehiscence, and stenosis. Proceedings of the American Thoracic Society. 2009;6:79-93

[47] Dutau H, Cavailles A, Sakr L, et al. A retrospective study of silicone stent placement for management of anastomotic airway complications in lung transplant recipients: Short- and long-term outcomes. The Journal of Heart and Lung Transplantation. 2010;29:658-664

[48] Wahidi MM, Ravenel J, Palmer SM, McAdams HP. Progression of idiopathic pulmonary fibrosis in native lungs after single lung transplantation. Chest. 2002;121:2072-2076

[49] Elicker BM, Golden JA, Ordovas KG, Leard L, Golden TR, Hays SR. Progression of native lung fibrosis in lung transplant recipients with idiopathic pulmonary fibrosis. Respiratory Medicine. 2010;104:426-433

[50] Frost AE, Keller CA, Noon GP, Short HD, Cagle PT. Outcome of the native lung after single lung transplant. Multiorgan Transplant Group. Chest. 1995;107:981-984

[51] Kim DS, Collard HR, King TE Jr. Classification and natural history of the idiopathic interstitial pneumonias. Proceedings of the American Thoracic Society. 2006;3:285-292

[52] Mathew J, Kratzke RA. Lung cancer and lung transplantation: A review. Journal of Thoracic Oncology. 2009;4:753-760

[53] Grignani G, Maiolo A. Cytokines and hemostasis. Haematologica. 2000;85:967-972

[54] Nathan SD, Barnett SD, Urban BA, Nowalk C, Moran BR, Burton N. Pulmonary embolism in idiopathic pulmonary fibrosis transplant recipients. Chest. 2003;123:1758-1763

[55] Burns KE, Iacono AT. Pulmonary embolism on postmortem examination: An under-recognized complication in lung-transplant recipients? Transplantation. 2004;77:692-698

[56] Kroshus TJ, Kshettry VR, Hertz MI, Bolman RM 3rd. Deep venous thrombosis and pulmonary embolism after lung transplantation. The Journal of Thoracic and Cardiovascular Surgery. 1995;110:540-544

[57] Hosenpud JD, Bennett LE, Keck BM, Edwards EB, Novick RJ. Effect of diagnosis on survival benefit of lung transplantation for end-stage lung disease. Lancet. 1998;351:24-27

[58] Thabut G, Christie JD, Ravaud P, et al. Survival after bilateral versus single lung transplantation for patients with chronic obstructive pulmonary disease: A retrospective analysis of registry data. Lancet. 2008;371:744-751

[59] Santana MJ, Feeny D, Jackson K, Weinkauf J, Lien D. Improvement in health-related quality of life after lung transplantation. Canadian Respiratory Journal. 2009;16:153-158

[60] Smeritschnig B, Jaksch P, Kocher A, et al. Quality of life after lung transplantation: A cross-sectional study. The Journal of Heart and Lung Transplantation. 2005;24:474-480

[61] Kugler C, Fischer S, Gottlieb J, et al. Health-related quality of life in two hundred-eighty lung transplant recipients. The Journal of Heart and Lung Transplantation. 2005;24:2262-2268

[62] Ortega T, Deulofeu R, Salamero P, et al. Health-related quality of life before and after a solid organ transplantation (kidney, liver, and lung) of four Catalonia hospitals. Transplantation Proceedings. 2009;41:2265-2267

Chapter 5

The Role of Pulmonary Rehabilitation in Patients with Idiopathic Pulmonary Fibrosis

Elena Dantes, Emanuela Tudorache
and Milena Adina Man

Abstract

Idiopathic pulmonary fibrosis (IPF) is known as one of the most severe lung conditions and the worst form of interstitial lung disease (ILD). There is a continuing concern about clinical research to identify new therapies that influence the quality of life in patients diagnosed with this chronic progressive pulmonary disease, with an average survival of 3–5 years. Although in recent years great progress has been made to slow down the functional decline of the disease with new antifibrotic therapies, it has failed to alter the prognosis and survival of IPF patients. Clinical trials and recent ATS/ERS guidelines have brought at least moderate and low levels of evidence for increased effort tolerance, decreased symptoms, and improved quality of life following participation in lung rehabilitation programs for ILD patients and in particular those with IPF. Pulmonary rehabilitation has been shown to be a standard of care for COPD patients, but their personalized application to patients with IPF has had positive short-term results, becoming a safe alternative to non-pharmacological treatment. The chapter includes the general objectives of rehabilitation programs, their type and structure, ways of complex assessment of patients before and after a training exercise, types of exercises, and short- and long-term results.

Keywords: idiopathic pulmonary fibrosis (IPF), pulmonary rehabilitation program (PRP), physical activity, exercise training, quality of life

1. Introduction

Idiopathic pulmonary fibrosis (IPF) is a chronic disease that affects exclusively the lung, with an unknown etiology and a fast-progressive irreversible evolution, therefore disabling the adult. For most of the patients, the average survival is approximately 3–5 years from diagnosis [1, 2]. With an unpredictable but progressive evolution (slower, stable, or accelerated decline from patient to patient), the disease is characterized by a chronic presence of symptoms, specifically the exertional dyspnea, low tolerance to effort, and the deterioration of the quality of life [1–4]. The diagnosis of the disease is often delayed and not reported until advanced stages [5]. A hope to halt the progression of the disease occurred with the demonstration of the reduction in the functional decline of the new pharmacological agents, pirfenidone and nintedanib, without claiming to cure the disease [1–5]. IPF remains a life-threatening illness in which the patient is fighting for survival as long as possible, striving to cope with the symptoms and the noticeable fatigue. Given that this is a fatal disease, some of the needs identified in patients with IPF and their families are easy access to information and IPF specialists, the existence of more treatment methods, emotional support, and access to end-of-life care [3].

The indication of pulmonary rehabilitation (PR) for patients with IPF came from the positive results stemming from the exercise training program (ETP) in COPD. Thus, numerous clinical studies performed on patients with IPF proved that their health and wellness could be improved, at least for short periods, through ETP which are personalized and supervised by specialists [2].

Pulmonary rehabilitation program (PRP) is an evidence-based recommendation for the non-pharmacological treatment of patients with chronic pulmonary diseases, especially for COPD, but also for interstitial lung diseases [1, 4]. PRP must be included in the integrative treatment of IPF, taking into consideration the severity of the disease, high mortality during exacerbations, a modest response to new drugs, and accelerated deterioration of lung function.

2. The indication of pulmonary rehabilitation starting from pathophysiology in IPF

The usual interstitial pneumonia (UIP) pattern (fibrosis with collagen and matrix deposition, the presence of fibroblastic foci and alveolar collapse, pulmonary heterogeneous architectural distortion and honeycombing presence) determines the main pathophysiological changes in IPF: loss of lung volume, decreased lung compliance, abnormal pulmonary gas exchange with oxygen diffusion limitation, low mixed venous oxygen content, circulatory impairments, and alveolar ventilation/perfusion ($V'A/Q'$) mismatching [6, 7].

Pulmonary function tests reveal restrictive pulmonary dysfunction, indirect signs of increased elastic recoil, and decrease in diffusion capacity for carbon monoxide (DLCO). Pulse oximetry and arterial blood gases reveal hypoxemia initially only during exercise and, in advanced cases, as well during resting [2, 7]. Patients with IPF have reduced maximal or peak oxygen uptake ($V'O_{2peak}$), peak work rate, and submaximal exercise endurance [7].

The progressive installation of morphophysiopathological changes is reflected in the clinical symptoms of patients. The exertional dyspnea is the first and most important symptom of IPF patients. The more advanced the disease, the more severe the dyspnea is. The patients tend to be less physically active and more depressed [8]. The level of dyspnea is strongly correlated with the exercise capacity, the quality of life, and mortality [1, 8, 9]. Other associated symptoms are fatigue, dry cough, chest discomfort, and leg pain. These symptoms are mild or inconsistent at the beginning of the disease, but they get worse over time and lead to an impairment of daily activities [10]. Symptomology and physical inactivity are directly related to depression, quality of life (QoL), and increased mortality [10, 11].

Consequently, the most important mechanisms that limit effort capacity and change the IPF patient's lifestyle, into a sedentary one, are inefficient breathing mechanics, abnormal pulmonary gas exchange, circulatory impairment, and exercise-induced hypoxemia [1, 7, 12, 13]. In time, progressive exercise-induced hypoxemia leads to respiratory and skeletal muscle dysfunction [1, 7]. Non-pharmacological interventions must take into account these mechanisms and create programs that seek to influence the patients' outcomes positively. PR is a safe and effective non-pharmacological treatment [14].

The official ERS/ARS statement define pulmonary rehabilitation as "Pulmonary rehabilitation is a comprehensive intervention based on a thorough patient assessment followed by patient tailored therapies that include, but are not limited to, exercise training, education, and behavior change, designed to improve the physical and psychological condition of people with chronic respiratory disease and to promote the long-term adherence to health-enhancing behaviors" [11].

PR decreases dyspnea, improves exercise capacity, and helps to cope with functional activities of daily life in IPF patients, even though the significance of these benefits is smaller and lasts for less time than in other chronic lung disease like COPD [15–20].

3. General objectives of pulmonary rehabilitation in IPF

- Decreasing symptoms, especially dyspnea

- Increasing effort capacity

- Enhancing the quality of life, health, and wellness

- Improving muscle strength and endurance

- Maintaining joint mobility

- Increasing tolerance to physical activity with the improved cardiometabolic and respiratory profile

- Improving well-being and cognitive functions

- Decreasing depression and anxiety

- Offer social and psychological support with the possibility of occupational and group therapy

- Promoting pro-healthy behaviors, with decreasing effort deconditioning

- Self-management of the disease [20–22]

The adaptation of pulmonary rehabilitation programs for IPF started from those applied to patients with COPD. It is advised to take into account the pathophysiology mechanisms particular to IPF and the clinical particularities of these patients. Patients have a respiratory pattern of frequent, superficial, and rapid breaths that worsen during exercise [7, 17, 18]. The frequent association of pulmonary hypertension (PH) aggravates the symptoms [1, 4]. An explanation for the positive results of PRP could be that repetitive ventilator stimulus during physical training sessions increases chest expansion and secondary pleural elasticity and pulmonary compliance while also improving V'A/Q' mismatch, increasing $V'O_{2peak}$ [13, 23]. Also, deep breathing exercises with stretching and the training of respiratory muscles, including the diaphragm, can help to reduce dyspnea [20, 23, 24].

4. Assessment of IPF patients before and after PRP

Before entering into a PRP, patients with IPF need to be assessed by the multidisciplinary team regarding clinical and functional status, imaging, effort tolerance, quality of life, physical activities of daily living (PADL), the presence of comorbidities, needs, and expectations from the pharmacological treatment. The evaluation of comorbidities such as coronary arterial disease, systemic and pulmonary hypertension, right and left ventricle dysfunction, and arrhythmias during exercise is critical. The additional impairment of the cardiovascular system decreases the effort capacity and worsens dyspnea and prognosis of patients [1, 2, 25]. This complex assessment also has the role in determining the type, intensity, and results of the PRP.

4.1 Symptoms assessment

Dyspnea is the most significant and disabling symptom for IPF patients. It can be objectively identified before, in the end, and at any time within PRP and can modulate the intensity of exercise. In studies targeting PR in IPF, dyspnea is quantified using one of the following scales:

4.1.1 Modified Medical Research Council (MMRC)

The *Modified Medical Research Council (MMRC)* scale is a well-known tool which assesses the dyspnea based on 5 degrees that are reported by the patient depending on his physical activity tolerance. It seems that dyspnea severity correlates with lung function parameters and Saint George Respiratory Questionnaire (SGRQ). The patient identifies the number that best matches his/her shortness of breath [26–28]. The standardized mean difference (SMD) for change in dyspnea in favor of exercise training (ET) is considered to be −0.66 (95% CI=1.05-0.28) [15]. MMRC dyspnea scales reflect the severity of the limitation of daily activity, pulmonary function, and quality of life and correlate with mortality. It can replace, where it is not possible to asses, the peripheral muscle strength, functional exercise capacity, and ADL performance [29].

4.1.2 University of California, San Diego Shortness of Breath Questionnaire (UCSD SOB)

The *University of California, San Diego Shortness of Breath Questionnaire (UCSD SOB)* uses a 24 questions questionnaire about the level of dyspnea during daily activities [30]. Five points represent a significant mean difference [31]. Dyspnea measured by UCSD SOB showed the strongest correlations with 6MWD [32].

4.1.3 Baseline Dyspnea Index (BDI)/Transition Dyspnea Index (TDI)

The *Baseline Dyspnea Index (BDI)/Transition Dyspnea Index (TDI)* assesses on a 5-degree scale (from 0 to 4), the daily dyspnea level in response to three categories of questions on functional impairment, the magnitude of task, and the magnitude of effort [26, 33, 34]. TDI records the changes from the initial value, the total score varying between −9 (worsening) and +9 (improvement). The significant minimal difference between TDI is 1 point [33, 34].

4.1.4 Modified Borg Scale (MBS)

The *Modified Borg Scale (MBS)* has 10 points (from 0 to 10), where participants choose descriptive terms that best suit their current state (0 = no dyspnea, 5 = moderate dyspnea, 10 = very severe dyspnea). It is used before and after performing a submaximal effort test such as 6MWT. The standardized significant mean difference (SMD) for change is 1 point [31]. During exercise training sessions in the PRP, the Borg scale is used as an essential tool to recommend workload [35].

It was shown that there are correlations between clinical dyspnea rating and exercise capacity, exercised gas exchange and exercise capacity, and SGRQ in patients with IPF [26, 29, 36].

4.2 Pulmonary function tests

Pulmonary function tests, including forced vital capacity (FVC), total lung capacity (TLC), maximal voluntary ventilation (FEV1 x 35), and diffusion capacity for carbon monoxide (DLCO), are important for stratifying the severity of the patient's condition, but generally, PRP does not significantly influence the results of these tests [20]. The severity of dysfunction may guide the type and intensity of physical exercise and may be a warning about the risk of adverse effects (severe hypoxemia, hypotension, arrhythmias, etc.)

4.3 Standardized effort tests

Standardized effort tests are important for choosing the intensity of training programs.

4.3.1 The 6-minute walking test (6MWT)

The 6-minute walking test (6MWT) is a simple and safe tool used for IPF patients, where the subject moves in his rhythm [37]. It is performed according to ATS guidelines in a 30-m corridor [38]. 20–30 min of rest is recommended before and after the 6MWD test. The blood pressure, heart rate, respiratory frequency, oxygen saturation (SpO_2), the severity of dyspnea, and fatigue are assessed by the modified Borg scale [38, 39]. SpO_2 is recorded in the sitting position. It is recommended that the 6MWD test be performed with a SpO_2 Holter, to record the length of the desaturation and the lowest value of oxygen [40]. It is always necessary to take into consideration the contraindications of walking tests and also the indications of interruption of the test. An important cessation criterion is a desaturation below 85% or tachycardia [80% of the theoretical maximum heart rate (220–age)], a situation easily met in IPF patients [1, 41]. The distance covered by the patient in 6 minutes is compared with the predicted value estimated by the formulas (women: 493 + (2.2 × height (cm)) − (0.93 × G (kg)) − 5.3 × age (years) and for the male + 17 m). The lower limit of normal 6MWD is the theoretical distance minus 100 m [42–44]. The 6-minute walk test distance (6MWD) does not correlate with sex, age, body mass index, and other medical comorbidities, but it is an independent predictor of survival rate, better than FVC and DLCO [37]. The 12-minute walk test is less used for IPF patients because it requires greater effort.

The minimal clinical important significant difference (MCID) for 6MWD varies with the author, but a change of approximately 30 m is considered to be significant in IPF patients [32, 41, 44, 45].

4.3.2 Cardiopulmonary exercise tests

Cardiopulmonary exercise tests, when available, provide details on the mechanisms of effort intolerance. Measures of the anaerobic threshold, peak oxygen consumption ($V'O_{2peak}$), and peak work rate (WR) are essential for determining the intensity of PRP and for assessing the benefits in dynamics. The SpO_2, blood pressure, and 12-lead electrocardiogram are also recorded during these tests [46]. Cardiopulmonary stress tests are the gold standard for assessing the effort intolerance due to either lung, cardiac, or musculoskeletal pathologies. It is performed with a cycle ergometer or treadmill, but there is also a portable metabolic device. Cycle ergometry is the preferred method of being safer, with few movement artifacts, allowing a constant increase in workload, and is slightly influenced by weight [46–48]. Treadmill testing involves a kind of effort more common to patient's daily activities (walking and running) and can train more muscle mass. Therefore, the $V'O_{2peak}$ is 5–10% higher than in cyclo-ergometry. Effort tests have a role in selecting patients for PRP and establishing rehabilitation design protocols, as well as evaluating outcomes [48].

In patients with advanced IPF, it is not always possible to perform cyclo-ergometry. Volitional fatigue or increased oxygen desaturation ($SpO_2 < 80\%$) is quickly reached, and dizziness or mental confusion may also occur within 10–12 min of effort [48]. The incremental exercise testing shows decreased aerobic capacity ($V'O_{2peak} \sim 62\%$ from predicted) and reduced maximal achievable workload in ILD. Other changes in IPF patients such as inefficient ventilation, desaturation, gas exchange abnormalities, circulator, and skeletal muscle dysfunction are reported [2]. These changes provoke a downward spiral of hypoxia, limited exercise capacity, deconditioning, shallow breathing pattern, and pulmonary hypertension [48].

4.4 Doppler-echocardiographic assessment

Doppler-echocardiographic assessment of pulmonary artery systolic pressure should be assessed because a significant percentage of the IPF patients develop PH from early stages of the disease [10, 49]. It represents an important prognostic parameter [10, 49]. It usually replaces right heart catheterization, echocardiography being a noninvasive and widely available tool for screening PH. A substantial desaturation during exercise or a disproportionate exercise limitation related to the degree of lung restriction will increase the suspicion of PH [7, 10].

4.5 Chest high-resolution computed tomography (HRCT) and lung ultrasound

HRCT is the essential method to diagnose IPF. If the HRCT shows a pattern of usual interstitial pneumonia (UIP), this being the most characteristic to IPF, then its presence avoids invasive procedure such as lung biopsy. In the last few years, radiation-free techniques, such as the lung ultrasound, appear to be very sensitive in detecting fibrotic change or monitoring disease progression [50]. Imaging on HRCT is important and significant before a PRP, but its rehabilitation benefits are not assessed according to the initial findings.

4.6 Physical activity of daily living (PADL)

Physical activity of daily living (PADL) has a major impact on the quality of life and well-being of IPF patients and needs to be evaluated. PADL refers to volunteer movements that the patient performs at home, during professional or recreational activities that are energy-consuming. There is an inversely proportional relationship between PADL and sedentariness, reduced autonomy, disability, risk of hospitalization, and death [51]. Besides, the disease severity (dyspnea levels, $SpO_2 < 88\%$, DLCO < 40%, 6MWD, the extent of honeycombing on computed tomography, level of PH) was associated with lower physical activity among patients' stable IPF [52].

4.6.1 PADL assessment

PADL assessment is performed either by direct observation (time and staff consuming because it is individually applied), energy expenditure (for research calorimetry), questionnaires, and other devices with motion sensors (detect movement and quantify PADL: pedometers, accelerometers, or physical activity monitors). The questionnaires are subjective methods of evaluating the effects of the symptoms on the patient's daily activities and quality of life, and they are instruments that are used in evaluating PRP [53]. Achieving progress through training programs can motivate the patient to pursue an active lifestyle for as long as possible. Pedometers measure only the distance covered daily (10,000 steps/day for a healthy lifestyle in the general population), but the effort intensity is better quantified by accelerometers [54]. These are preferred in sedentary or disabled patients, being more sensitive to the detection and description of movements. Daily activity can be quantified using the activity monitor for at least seven consecutive days from awakening to bed [2]. The intensity of physical activity is evaluated on a scale of 1–5, depending on the energy expenditure, expressed in the metabolic equivalent task (METS) [55].

4.6.2 The questionnaires used in PADL evaluation

The questionnaires used in PADL evaluation for IPF are easy to apply, cheap, self-administered, validated (internal consistency and test-retest reliability) and correlate with the estimated energy consumption by the methods mentioned above. The most commonly used questionnaires in clinical studies, which are extrapolated to IPF patients, are as follows:

4.6.2.1 Self-report 7-day short form International Physical Activity Questionnaire (IPAQ)

Self-report 7-day short form International Physical Activity Questionnaire (IPAQ) [2, 56] consists of nine items which evaluate the level of physical activity that is quantified in METS for the effort intensity: vigorous (8 METS), moderate (4 METS), walking (3.3 METS), and sitting times. The total score is the sum of all types of activities (the number of minutes spent/day) multiplied by the level of energy (MET) and multiplied by the amount of time spent/week [(MET)-min/week] [55]. An active patient is considered to perform 600 METS-min/week (150 min/week × 4METS moderate intensity activity) [54, 57]. IPAQ $\leq$ 417 (MET-min/week) $\Delta SpO_2 < 10$ (%) represents the cutoff which predicts mortality in patients with IPF [2]. However, there were differences between the self-reported patient score on the questionnaire and the accelerometer's results, depending on sex, age, education level, and body mass index (BMI). There is also a short form for this IPAQ [58].

4.6.2.2 Barthel index (BI)

Barthel index (BI) is based on basic physical activities for self-grooming, such as feeding, toilet use, bladder and bowel control, walking, dressing, bathing, brushing, or ascending and descending stairs. The total scores vary between 0 and 70; higher scores are associated with more active subjects. A change in the BI score after 1 month of ET4 was arbitrarily classified as mild (a decrease of <10 points), moderate (10–15 points), or severe (>15 points) [59]. This index reflects the independence levels in PADL in IPF patients.

4.6.2.3 Baecke questionnaire

In *Baecke questionnaire*, the score reflects the level of energy consumed performing professional activities, sports, and entertainment and is also adapted for the elderly, obese, and Parkinson's disease or cardiovascular patients [60].

4.6.2.4 *Stanford Seven-Day Physical Activity and Stanford Usual Activity questionnaires*

Stanford Seven-Day Physical Activity and Stanford Usual Activity questionnaires are applied during an interview. The first one relates to the time spent doing physical activities and sleeping for the past 7 days. The second focuses on moderate and intense activities in the last 3 months [61].

The PADL level is positively influenced by supervised PRP that lasts at least 7–8 weeks.

4.7 The quality of life questionnaire

The quality of life questionnaire has been developed and validated extrapolating those applied to COPD patients, given the lack of a specific disease-specific questionnaire for IPF [56].

4.7.1 *St. George Respiratory Questionnaire (SGRQ)*

St. George Respiratory Questionnaire and St. George Respiratory Questionnaire IPF-specific version (SGRQ-I) consist of 50 items referring to three categories: symptoms (8 items), activity (16 items), and impact (26 items) [36, 62, 63]. The total score varies from 0 to 100 points. Higher scores reveal a poorer health-related quality of life. SGRQ-I is reliable and comparable to the original SGRQ [64]. The SGRQ score was significantly correlated with FVC, FEV1 (%), 6MWD, and MRC. On the other hand, it did not show a significant correlation with DLCO or the level of desaturation at 6MWD, compared with CAT questionnaire [64].

4.7.2 *Medical Outcomes Short-Form 36 (SF-36)*

Medical Outcomes Short-Form 36 (SF-36) is a generic health-related quality of life questionnaire. It consists of eight multidimension items as general health, vitalities, physical functioning, physical role/problems, body pain, emotional roles/problems, social functioning, and mental health. Each of the dimensions is scored from 0 to 100. Higher scores indicate a better health-related quality of life [65].

4.7.3 *Hospital Anxiety and Depression Scale (HADS)*

The *Hospital Anxiety and Depression Scale (HADS)* can be applied in any disabling chronic disease which leads to impairment of the psychic/emotional status of patients [66].

4.7.4 *The Chronic Respiratory Disease Questionnaire (CRDQ)*

The Chronic Respiratory Disease Questionnaire (CRDQ) refers to dyspnea, fatigability, emotional impact, and self-control [67].

4.7.5 *COPD assessment test (CAT)*

COPD assessment test (CAT) was compared with other instruments applied to patients with IPF showing good psychometric properties among ILD patients. It is a self-administered questionnaire with eight items, each scored on a scale from 1 to 5. There is a strong correlation between the CAT score and SGRQ score, indicating that it can be used for health-related quality of life assessment among patients with

IPF. Furthermore, CAT showed higher correlations with the physiological parameters than the SGRQ [67].

4.7.6 Tool to Assess Quality of Life in Idiopathic Fibrosis (ATAQ-IPF)

The *Tool to Assess Quality of Life in Idiopathic Fibrosis (ATAQ-IPF)* is an extensive, 74 items, a disease-specific instrument which measures the symptoms adequately, sleep, emotions, relationships, therapies, finances, and many others. The score correlates with disease severity, but future studies are needed [8].

4.7.7 King's Brief Interstitial Lung Disease (K-BILD)

The *King's Brief Interstitial Lung Disease (K-BILD)* questionnaire is a validated and responsive questionnaire for longitudinal assessment of ILD patients' quality of life. A score change of 5 units is significant [68].

4.8 Muscle strength assessment

In muscle strength assessment, types of muscular impairment refer to mass (of different anatomical sites: biceps, triceps, etc.), strength, endurance, and performance [69]. Peripheral muscle force measurement may be important in PRP for understanding the impact of the disease on muscle mass, identifying patients at risk for physical impairment, and identifying those who can benefit from the prescription of an individualized resistance training program. Peripheral muscular dysfunction is a consequence of sedentary lifestyle, adopted by patients to avoid the symptoms and systemic effects of the disease (inflammation, hypoxemia, nutritional deficiency, corticosteroid side effects, electrolyte imbalances). Commonly, quadriceps muscle dysfunction is used for the assessment of peripheral muscle strength. The tests that are used may be volitional (volitional techniques: identification of the maximum weight that the patient can lift, manual muscle testing with MRC scale, or by dynamometers: handheld and computerized) or non-volitional (electrical stimulation of involuntary muscle contraction). The quadriceps maximal isometric voluntary contraction (QMVC) or predictive formulas (different equations for predicting quadriceps muscle strength) are described in literature, especially in studies on patients with COPD [70–72]. It is considered that patients have quadriceps muscle weakness if the value is <80% of predicted [73]. Knee extensor and elbow flexor strength could be measured with handheld dynamometer [69].

5. Correlation between exercise tolerance, daily physical activity, and survival rate

a. **6MWD** is an independent and discriminating predictor of mortality among patients with IPF, more accurate than FVC or DLCO [74, 75]:

- Basal value <250 m correlates with twofold increase in mortality, and if it is less than 207 m, patients have a more than fourfold greater mortality rate.

- A decrease of $SpO_2 < 88\%$ during 6MWT is marker for increased mortality.

- A decrease in the walking distance within 6 months, greater than 50 m, would increase the mortality rate by three times.

- A delayed heart rate return in 1 minute after the end of the 6MWD test and a variation <13 beats/min are strongly correlated with increased mortality.

b. **Daily life physical activity level** [76–78]:

- IPF patients are highly sedentary, having a daily physical activity level which is 35% lower than healthy sedentary controls.

- A value under 3.287 steps/day on accelerometers was associated with a poorer prognosis and three times higher risk for death for IPF patients.

- Peripheral muscle dysfunction related with a decrease of the physical activity level of daily life and exercise limitation is associated with reduced survival.

6. Types of pulmonary rehabilitation programs

PRP for IPF patients include several types of exercises, such as aerobic, resistance, flexibility, balance training, and respiration technique. Their selection is based on the everyday lifestyle of each patient, preferences, disease severity, and the advantages of where the PRP will take place:

- "Inpatient" rehabilitation centers are a more appropriate method for the supervised exercise programs taking into account the symptoms and the risk of severe effort desaturation that may occur. The advantage is that during exercise sessions, patients are monitored for blood pressure, heart rate, SpO_2, and symptoms, and the urgent treatment is available in case of complications [79, 80].

- "Outpatient"-based programs take place in the patient's home under the assistance of a healthcare professional with expertise in exercise training.

- *Home-based rehabilitation* programs are an alternative to in-/outpatient programs. They are easy to perform, practical, cheap, and equally as effective, but unfortunately have a lower adherence rate and less improvements, so it is necessary to be supervised by phone calls [12, 78, 79, 81].

- Combined programs start in a specialized structure and continues at home after the patients are familiar with the type and intensity of exercise [83].

PRP includes physical training, patient education, and nutritional and psychological support [11]. Regardless of the type of PRP, it is beneficial to start it as soon as possible. We will keep in mind that the intensity of rehabilitation depends on the severity of functional impairment and is personalized to each patient. The physical therapist starts from breath retraining and relaxing postures which increase chest expansion and relax the inspiratory muscles (Jacobson, Schultz technique). They reinforce proper breathing patterns (diaphragm) and include exercises that tonify respiratory and skeletal muscle (endurance and resistance) in order to increase patients' exercise capacity [2].

7. Types of exercises

The main objective of these training programs is teaching patients how to perform a series of structured and repetitive exercises that improve or maintain their physical fitness and decrease the respiratory discomfort [82].

Educating patients about pursuing an active lifestyle even in the presence of IPF should be based on information about the types of exercises that can be performed, the regularity and duration of each session, and general instructions on how and what to follow through the program. During the follow-up with their patients, the doctor may be confronted with various questions, doubts, and anxiety from the patients. In the early stages of the disease, when the symptoms are not disabling, the patient's motivation to follow a PRP is low. In advanced stages, the motivation is stronger because dyspnea limits exercise capacity and daily activities. According to several studies, the PRP with greatest benefits have 6–12 weeks programs, with 2–3 sessions per week of 30 minutes duration. The exercise intensity is determined by patients' walking speed on 6MWD (starting at 70–80%), or by the maximum workload on cycle ergometer test (50–60% or more of peak WR on CPET for cycling), maximum heart rate (up to 80%), or on the intensity of symptoms on the Borg scale (to reach a score above 5–7). The effort intensity can also be calculated from an average heart rate ± 5 beats, obtained in the last 3 minutes of the effort test [2, 21, 33, 84].

A comprehensive training program should include several types of exercises: breathing and balance exercises, aerobic, endurance, and flexibility (stretching) [2, 12, 20, 33, 84].

For increasing the endurance to effort, aerobic exercises can be used to train different muscle groups, depending on the patients' preferences and physical resources. Aerobic exercises can include walking, stair climbing, treadmill walking, leg cycling, semi-recumbent cycling, or step climbing on an ergometer adapted for lower limbs [16]. Resistance training refers to the increase in muscle strength and can be achieved by performing repeated exercises for upper and lower limbs, arm raising, knee-extension, sit-to-stand, and strength training using elastic bands. In these types of exercises, the muscles work against an external force applied by a device from the physiotherapy room or against their own body weight. They can also use weights. These exercises are grouped in 2–4 sets, with 10–15 repetitions, followed by breaks of 45–60 s. Each set of exercises targets specific muscle groups [85]. These exercises are recommended due to the fact that IPF patients have reduced muscle mass, strength, and endurance, compared with healthy subjects. They develop atrophy and muscle weakness, especially in lower limbs [86, 87]. Stretching exercises are activities designed to maintain or increase joint mobility and muscle relaxation. Strength training targets major muscle groups of the upper and lower body. There is a wide range of exercises that could be applied by physiotherapist [88]:

- Shoulder wheel

- Multiple movements of shoulder by changing his position as abduction, externally rotates the shoulder, flexion, and extension

- Sitting or standing biceps curls

- Mid-back rowing

- Shoulder flexion or extension

- Sitting or standing chest presses and triceps extensions

- Lower body exercises: standing hip abduction and extension

- Seated knee flexion and extension

- Internal and external rotations of the abducted shoulder with the elbow flexed 90 degrees

- Wall push-ups

- Chair squat

- Dumbbells shoulder press

- Dumbbells biceps curls

- Dumbbells arm extension

- Abdominal curl-ups

- Seated single leg hamstring stretch

- Standing quadriceps stretch

- Chest stretch

- Overhead reach stretch and wall cat stretch

For strength training there are three types of therapeutic bands that can be used: yellow, followed by red, and then green.

Respiratory muscle training or breathing exercises are extremely important, especially for patients with advanced disease, because they focus on diaphragm training, by teaching patients abdominal breathing techniques [79, 89].

There are no strictly standardized protocols for the PRP, allowing an experienced physiotherapist to tailor the patient's training structure in order to maximize the benefits.

The structure of a rehabilitation program should be seen as a multistage process:

- Firstly, the patient learns different types of exercise and different techniques, which can be divided into four categories (aerobic, endurance, flexibility, and breathing). Their intensity should be adapted to the severity of patient's pulmonary impairment, typically 50–60% of the work peak rate for aerobic exercise and 70–80% of the walking speed in 6MWT for endurance exercises (bicycle, treadmill, walking). The program can start with breathing exercises or balance training, continued by aerobic exercise and resistance training. Exercises should primarily focus on increasing the strength and the muscle mass of the lower limbs and diaphragm. The interval technique can also be used, allowing the patient to rest between exercises. In patients who experience desaturations ($SpO_2 < 85\%$) during training, oxygen supplementation should be considered in order to maintain SpO_2 above 88% [21]. During a program of 2–3 sessions/week, for 4–6 weeks, under the supervision of a physiotherapist, a patient can learn and become adequately trained to pass into the second phase.

- In the continuation and improvement phase, subjects can progressively increase both the frequency (3–4 times/week), duration, and intensity of the sessions. The aerobic program can be extended to 20–50 min and can be performed at an intensity of 60–85% of the work peak rate. The resistance training can last between 20 and 30 min, with an intensity of 80–100% from the average walking speed obtained in the 6MWD test. Also, the programs recommend including 10–15 min of stretching and a minimum of 5 min of diaphragmatic or pursed lip breathing [90].

- The maintenance phase is important for preserving the benefits of a PRP, for decreasing the anxiety and depression level, and for increasing the quality of life. It is recommended to maintain the types and the intensity of exercises that will lead to a level of fatigue between 5 and 7 on the Borg scale.

Each patient should be reassessed at 3–6 months, in terms of effort tolerance, quality of life, disease progression, and response to pharmacological treatment.

In brief, a supervised training program for patients with IPF should recommend:

- 4–6 weeks, 2–3 sessions/week

- Aerobic effort 20–40 min

- Stretching 10–15 min

- Breathing techniques 5–10 min

- Adjusting the work intensity so it can be tolerable for the patient

- Oxygen supplementation for patients who desaturate (SpO_2 85–88%)

- Intervals between exercises allowing better oxygenation

- Patient reassessment at the end of the 6 weeks

In a comprehensive PRP, patient's education begins from understanding the patient's needs and providing detailed information regarding the nature and expected course of the disease, solutions for symptoms management, benefits and side effects of treatments (depression, anxiety, obesity, diabetes, cardiovascular disease), the indication of oxygen supplementation, energy conservation techniques, relaxation and recreation methods, stress management, coping techniques for anxiety and depression, smoking cessation, and solutions for the improvement of quality of life. Medical education sessions usually precede exercise training sessions. This will be individualized for each patient, ensuring optimal communication between the patient and the multidisciplinary team. Educational assessment begins with the identification of difficulties, focusing on the change of the health-related behavior. Goals need to be established in the short, medium, and long term, to increase the patient's motivation to follow a PRP. Educational therapy plays a role in the relief of symptoms and quality of life improvement, optimizing the benefits of a PRP [11].

Nutritional support refers to weight control and a balanced diet, with obesity or weight loss being associated with a poor prognosis. Adipose mass can be evaluated pre- and post-PR, using different skinfold calipers for the analysis of body composition by skinfold thickness measurements [91].

Due to the life-threatening course of the disease, the psychological support should be considered for each patient. The dialog among the patient, the patient's family, and healthcare professionals can decrease the depression and anxiety in more than 50% of ILD patients [56].

8. Results of the exercise training programs

Studies conducted support the beneficial effects of PR programs, at the end of which patients with IPF present [15, 19, 33]:

- Improvement in functional capacity

- Improvement in 6MWD results over SMD: 35.63 m (95% CI 16.02–55.23 m)

- Improvement in $V'O_2$ peak at 6WMD 1.46 mL/kg/min^{-1} (95% CI 0.54–2.39 mL/kg/min^{-1})

- Increased physical activity levels (IPAQ)

- Significant reduction in dyspnea: SMD −0.68 (95% CI −1.12 to −0.25)

- Improvement in wellness and health-related quality of life, especially for those with severe disease SMD 0.59 (95% CI 0.14–1.03)

- Increased muscular fitness

Quality of the evidence regarding the impact of PR programs in IPF patients after Dowman et al. [15]:

1. Change in 6-min walk distance—moderate ⊕⊕⊕⊖

2. Change in $V'O_2$ peak uptake at cardiopulmonary exercise test—low ⊕⊕⊖⊖

3. Change in maximum ventilation cardiopulmonary exercise test—low ⊕⊕⊖⊖

4. Change in dyspnea score MMRC Dyspnea Scale—low ⊕⊕⊖⊖

5. Change in quality of life CRDQ (total score)—low ⊕⊕⊖⊖

6. Month survival—low ⊕⊕⊖⊖

A follow-up was performed 8–12 weeks after end of rehabilitation.

The review used the Grades of Recommendation, Assessment, Development and Evaluation (GRADE) to evaluate the study results: "Moderate quality: Further research is likely to have an important impact on our confidence in the estimate of effect and may change the estimate. Low quality: Further research is very likely to have an important impact on our confidence in the estimate of effect and is likely to change the estimate" [15].

The increase in effort capacity is directly related to training frequency, three to five sessions per week being optimal and fewer than two sessions being unlikely to produce meaningful change [92].

It is considered that a PR has been beneficial if there has been an increase of more than 50 m at 6MWD test (31–81 m gained in PR in different clinical trials) and a minimum amount of physical activity at 200 METS-min/week [10 min × 4METS (moderate intensity in the IPAQ questionnaire) × 5 times/week. Longer programs and more frequent sessions (12 or more) appear to have a greater benefit; however these benefits can be lost after 3–6 months, if the training does not continue and patients fail to maintain an active lifestyle [11]. There are discrepancies in the outcome of the studies, in patients who have undergone a pulmonary rehabilitation program, discussing the responder or non-responder label depending on whether or not the walking distance of 6MWD or $V'O_2$ has improved. Non-responders are considered patients whose result of 6MWT did not rise above or equal to 30 m after PR (30 m considered as MCID) [93]. Also, the responders had FEV1 and TLC raised after the rehabilitation program and significantly increased $V'O_2$ peak, carbon dioxide output (VCO_2), and minute ventilation (VE) in the 6MWT post-PR test, while non-responders showed greater desaturation during exercise [93].

The different results of the studies can be explained by:

- Training programs with differences in intensity, duration, and type of administration (inpatient/outpatient, supervised/unsupervised)

- Small numbers of participants

- Methodological limitation: methods of randomization (uncontrolled studies or nonrandomized, unblinded study)

- Limitations of retrospective studies

- Different control batches (other types of ILD, sham, etc.)

- Patients entering PR at different stages of severity

- Inclusion and exclusion criteria

- No follow-up data after exercise training

- Different outcomes

9. Lung transplant pre- and post-rehabilitation programs

Conforming to the International Society for Heart and Lung Transplantation (ISHLT), this pulmonary transplantation is performed for a variety of advanced lung diseases, IPF, together with COPD, being the most common indication. However, in posttransplant survival, IPF is associated with the worst prognosis. For patients with IPF, transplantation and supplemental oxygen were the only treatments strongly recommended by the latest ATS consensus document. A transplant discussion is recommended from the moment the positive diagnosis is confirmed due to low survival [94, 95].

Medical and surgical interventions in transplants have progressed in the last few years. All of these lead to a changing demographic of patients undergoing lung transplantation, including older subjects with multiple comorbidities, respiratory failure, and even those who require bridging to transplantation [95]. To ensure a high rate of posttransplant survival, both in the short and long term, these patients must be physically and psychologically trained for this complex process. PRP plays an essential role in pulmonary transplantation, both by optimizing physical function prior to surgical intervention and by facilitating posttransplant recovery. Although these PRP are mandatory in most transplant centers, to date there is no international pulmonary rehabilitation guideline for this patient category [95].

Physiotherapists working with lung transplant candidates and recipients need expertise both in general exercise training principles and in pre- and posttransplant rehabilitation, complications, oxygen titration, and side effects of medications. They should be able to adapt exercise programs according to the lung function changes and according to episodic illnesses (exacerbation) [95, 96].

Prior to transplant, patients should attend PRP and benefit from exercise training, aerobic, resistance, and flexibility, with or without oxygen support, in the tolerance limit. In early posttransplant period, mobility is advised even in ICU and in acute hospitalization, for the progression to independent function (transfers, walking, self-care, climbing stairs). In the next phase (1–6 month), they should gradually perform balance training, aerobic, resistance, and flexibility exercises, as tolerated. Oxygen can be supplemented to support exercise. In the long term (>6 months), patients should be included in home and community PR programs for maintaining and improving the benefits of this intervention [96]. All these aspects are the premises for a better prognosis and lower costs for the healthcare system.

10. General recommendations

- A multidisciplinary team that includes a respiratory specialist and a clinical psychotherapist should manage and supervise the inclusion in a PR program of patients with IPF and the structure and monitoring of the patients' exercise training sessions.

- In patients with severe IPF, it is preferred that programs are held in the hospital. In case programs are held at patient's home, then high-intensity exercises that could lead to desaturation and worsening of symptoms should be avoided.

- For long-term benefits, three to five sessions per week for a minimum of 6 weeks are optimal, less than two sessions being unlikely to produce significant change [92].

- Initially, the interval training method is preferred, and in time, the duration of the exercises can be increased. A break and rest are mandatory when excessive fatigue and dyspnea appear [12].

- The overall load increases gradually according to patient's tolerance, the intensity of effort being adjusted to patients' fatigue tolerance.

- Additional oxygen can be used during exercise as it allows for an increased endurance and intensity of exercise levels [1].

- Factors such as self-motivation, fear of adverse events, or comprehension may affect the ability to tolerate exercise training.

11. Conclusions

The pulmonary rehabilitation has become a clear indication as a non-pharmacological therapy for patients diagnosed with IPF. The benefits of pulmonary rehabilitation programs are reduced respiratory symptoms, especially dyspnea, and increased exercise tolerance and level of physical activity. All these lead to a lower level of anxiety and depression and therefore increased quality of life. These benefits are sustained in short term, 3–6 months. They can be maintained for a longer period if the patient has a responsible behavior and an active lifestyle.

Author details

Elena Dantes[1*], Emanuela Tudorache[2] and Milena Adina Man[3]

1 4th Clinical Department, Medicine Faculty, "Ovidius" University of Constanta, Pneumology Clinical Hospital, Romania

2 Department of Pulmonology, "Victor Babeş" University of Medicine and Pharmacy, Timisoara, Romania

3 Department of Pulmonology, "Iuliu Hatieganu" University of Medicine and Pharmacy, Cluj, Romania

*Address all correspondence to: elena.dantes@gmail.com

IntechOpen

References

[1] Raghu G, Collard HR, Egan JJ, Martinez FJ, Behr J, Brown KK, et al. An Official ATS/ERS/JRS/ALAT Statement: Idiopathic pulmonary fibrosis: Evidence-based guidelines for diagnosis and management. American Journal of Respiratory and Critical Care Medicine. 2011;**183**:788-824. DOI: 10.1164/rccm.2009-040GL

[2] Vainshelboim B. Exercise training in idiopathic pulmonary fibrosis: Is it of benefit? Breathe. 2016;**12**:130-138. DOI: 10.1183/20734735.006916

[3] Bonella F, Wijsenbeek M, Molina-Molina M, Duck A, Mele R, Geissler K, et al. European IPF patient charter: Unmet needs and a call to action for healthcare policymakers. The European Respiratory Journal. 2016;**47**:597-606. DOI: 10.1183/13993003.01204-2015

[4] Oancea C, Tudorache V. Pulmonary rehabilitation in interstitial lung disease. In: Strambu I et al., editors. Published by Romanian Pneumology Society. Diagnosis and Treatment Guide for Diffuse Interstitial Pneumopathies. 1st ed. Bucuresti; 2015. pp. 147-149. ISBN: 978-973-0-20120-8

[5] Strambu I, Salmen T, Traila D, Croitoru A. Romanian Registry for interstitial lung diseases (REGIS): Inclusion of patients in 3 years. European Respiratory Journal. 2017;**50**:PA868. DOI: 10.1183/1393003.congress-2017.PA868

[6] Kropski JA, Lawson WE, Young LR, Blackwell TS. Genetic studies provide clues on the pathogenesis of idiopathic pulmonary fibrosis. Disease Models & Mechanisms. 2013;**6**:9-17. DOI: 10.1242/dmm.010736

[7] Holland AE. Exercise limitation in interstitial lung disease—Mechanisms, significance and therapeutic options. Chronic Respiratory Disease. 2010;**7**:101-111. DOI: 10.1177/1479972309354689

[8] Swigris JJ, Kuschner WG, Jacobs SS, Wilson SR, Gould MK. Health-related quality of life in patients with idiopathic pulmonary fibrosis: A systematic review. Thorax. 2005;**60**:588-594. DOI: 10.1136/thx.2004.035220

[9] Mura M, Porretta MA, Bargagli E, Sergiacomi G, Zompatori M, Sverzellati N, et al. Predicting survival in newly diagnosed idiopathic pulmonary fibrosis: A 3-year prospective study. The European Respiratory Journal. 2012;**40**:101-109. DOI: 10.1183/09031936.00106011

[10] Meltzer EB, Noble PW. Idiopathic pulmonary fibrosis. Orphanet Journal of Rare Diseases. 2008;**3**:8. DOI: 10.1186/1750-1172-3-8

[11] Spruit MA, Singh SJ, Garvey C, ZuWallack R, Nici L, Rochester C, et al. An official American Thoracic Society/European Respiratory Society statement: Key concepts and advances in pulmonary rehabilitation. American Journal of Respiratory and Critical Care Medicine. 2013;**188**:e13-e64. DOI: 10.1164/rccm.201309-1634ST

[12] Ozalevli S, Karaali HK, Ilgin D, Ucan ES. Effect of home-based pulmonary rehabilitation in patients with idiopathic pulmonary fibrosis. Multidisciplinary Respiratory Medicine. 2010;**5**:31-37. DOI: 10.1186/2049-6958-5-1-31

[13] Lama VN, Martinez FJ. Resting and exercise physiology in interstitial lung diseases. Clinics in Chest Medicine. 2004;**25**:435-453. DOI: 10.1016/j.ccm.2004.05.005

[14] Fereira A, Garvey C, Connors GL, Hilling L, Rigler J, Farrell S, et al. Pulmonary rehabilitation in interstitial

lung disease. Benefits and predictors of response. Chest. 2009;**135**:442-447. DOI: 10.1378/chest.08-1458

[15] Dowman L, Hill CJ, Holland AE. Pulmonary rehabilitation for interstitial lung disease. Cochrane Database of Systematic Reviews. 2014;**10**:CD006322. DOI: 10.1002/14651858.CD006322.pub3

[16] Lacasse Y, Goldstein R, Lasserson TJ, Martin S. Pulmonary rehabilitation for chronic obstructive pulmonary disease. Cochrane Database of Systematic Reviews. 2006;**4**. DOI: 10.1002/14651858.CD003793.pub2

[17] Holland AE, Hill CJ, Conron M, Munro P, McDonald CF. Small changes in six-minute walk distance are important in diffuse parenchymal lung disease. Respiratory Medicine. 2009;**103**:1430-1435. DOI: 10.1016/j.rmed.2009.04.024

[18] Garvey C. Interstitial lung disease and pulmonary rehabilitation. Journal of Cardiopulmonary Rehabilitation and Prevention. 2010;**30**(3):141-146. DOI: 10.1097/HCR.0b013e3181c56b66

[19] Holland AE, Hill CJ, Glaspole I, Goh N, McDonald CF. Predictors of benefit following pulmonary rehabilitation for interstitial lung disease. Respiratory Medicine. 2012;**106**:429-435. DOI: 10.1016/j.rmed.2011.11.014

[20] Vainshelboim B, Oliveira J, Yehoshua L, Weiss I, Fox BD, Fruchter O, et al. Exercise training-based pulmonary rehabilitation program is clinically beneficial for idiopathic pulmonary fibrosis. Respiration. 2014;**88**:378-388. DOI: 10.1159/000367899

[21] Nakazawa A, Cox NS, Holland AE. Current best practice in rehabilitation in interstitial lung disease. Therapeutic Advances in Respiratory Disease. 2017;**11**(2):115-128. DOI: 10.1177/1753465816676048

[22] Nelson ME, Rejeski WJ, Blair SN, Duncan PV, Judge JO. Physical activity and public health in older adults: Recommendation from the American College of Sports Medicine and the American Heart Association. Circulation. 2007;**116**:1094-1105. DOI: 10.1161/CIRCULATIONAHA.107.185650

[23] American Thoracic Society. Idiopathic pulmonary fibrosis: Diagnosis and treatment. International consensus statement. American Thoracic Society (ATS), and the European Respiratory Society (ERS). American Journal of Respiratory and Critical Care Medicine. 2000;**161**:646-664. DOI: 10.1164/ajrccm.161.2.ats3-00

[24] Kenn K, Gloeckl R, Behr J. Pulmonary rehabilitation in patients with idiopathic pulmonary fibrosis—A review. Respiration. 2013;**86**:89-99. DOI: 10.1159/000354112

[25] Vainshelboim B, Kramer MR, Fox BD, Izhakian S, Sagie A, Oliveira J. Supervised exercise training improves exercise cardio-vascular function in idiopathic pulmonary fibrosis. European Journal of Physical and Rehabilitation Medicine. 2017;**53**:209-218. DOI: 10.23736/S1973-9087.16.04319-7

[26] Mahler DA, Harver A, Rosiello R, Daubenspeck JA. Measurement of respiratory sensation in interstitial lung disease. Evaluation of clinical dyspnea ratings and magnitude scaling. Chest. 1989;**96**:767-771. DOI: 10.1378/chest.96.4.767

[27] Papiris SA, Daniil ZD, Malagari K, Ries AL, Kaplan RM. The Medical Research Council dyspnea scale in the estimation of disease severity in idiopathic pulmonary fibrosis. Respiratory Medicine. 2005;**99**:755-761. DOI:10.1016/j.med.2004.10.018

[28] Bestall JC, Paul EA, Garrod R, Gamham R, Jines P, Wedzicha J. Usefulness of the Medical Research

Council (MRC) dyspnoea scale as a measure of disability in patients with chronic obstructive pulmonary disease. Thorax. 1999;**54**:581-586. DOI: 10.1136/thx.54.7.581

[29] Mahler DA, Weinberg DH, Wells CK, Feinstein AR. The measurement of dyspnea. Contents, interobserver agreement, and physiologic correlates of two new clinical indexes. Chest. 1984;**85**:751-758. DOI: 10.1378/chest.85.6.751

[30] Eakin EG, Resnikoff PM, Prewitt LM, Ries AL, Kaplan RM. Validation of a new dyspnea measure. The UCSD Shortness of Breath Questionnaire. Chest. 1998;**113**:619-624. DOI: 10.1378/chest.113.3.619

[31] Ries AL. Minimally clinically important difference for the UCSD shortness of breath questionnaire, Borg scale, and visual analog scale. COPD. 2005;**2**:105-110. DOI: 10.1081/COPD-200050655

[32] Nathan SD, du Bois RM, Albera C, Bradford WZ, Costabel U, Kartashov A, et al. Validation of test performance characteristics and minimal clinically important difference of the 6-minute walk test in patients with idiopathic pulmonary fibrosis. Respiratory Medicine. 2015;**109**:914-922. DOI: 10.1016/j.rmed.2015.04.008

[33] Nishiyama O, Kondoh Y, Kimura T, Kato K, Kataoka K, Ogawa T, et al. Effects of pulmonary rehabilitation in patients with idiopathic pulmonary fibrosis. Respirology. 2008;**13**:394-399. DOI: 10.1111/j.1440-1843.2007.01205.x

[34] Mahler DA, Witek TJ Jr. The MCID of the transition dyspnea index is a total score of one unit. COPD. 2005;**2**:99-103. DOI: 10.1081/COPD-200050666

[35] Chida M, Inase N, Ichioka M, Miyazato I, Marumo F. Ratings of perceived exertion in chronic obstructive pulmonary disease: A possible indicator for exercise training in patients with this disease. European Journal of Applied Physiology and Occupational Physiology. 1991;**62**:390-393. DOI: 10.1007/BF00626608

[36] Jones PW, Quirk FH, Baveystock CM. The St George's respiratory questionnaire. Respiratory Medicine. 1991;**85**:25-31. DOI: 10.1016/S0954-6111(06)80166-6

[37] Lederer DJ, Arcasoy SM, Wilt JS, D'Ovidio F, Sonett JR, Kawut SM. Six-minute-walk distance predicts waiting list survival in idiopathic pulmonary fibrosis. American Journal of Respiratory and Critical Care Medicine. 2006;**174**:659-664. DOI: 10.1164/rccm.200604-520OC

[38] ATS Committee on Proficiency Standards for Clinical Pulmonary Function Laboratories. ATS statement: Guidelines for the six-minute walk test. American Journal of Respiratory and Critical Care Medicine. 2002;**166**(1):111-117. DOI: 10.1164/ajrccm.166.1.at1102

[39] Rikli RE, Jones CJ. In: JMB Hughes, NB Pride, Champaign Jones PW, editors. The Senior Fitness Test Manual. Human Kinetics, Measurements of Breathlessness. Lung Function Test; 2000. WB SSaunders

[40] Mahler DA, Wells CK. Evaluation of Clinical Methods for Dyspnea Rating. Chest. 1988;**93**:580-586. DOI: 10.1378/chest.93.3.580

[41] Holland AE, Hill CJ, Conron M, Munro P, McDonald CF. Short-term improvement in exercise capacity and symptoms following exercise training in interstitial lung disease. Thorax. 2008;**63**:549-554. DOI: 10.1136/thx.2007.088070

[42] Enright PL, McBurnie MA, Bittner V, Tracy RP, McNamara R, Arnold A,

et al. The 6-min walk test. A quick measure of functional status in elderly adults. Chest. 2003;**123**(2):387-398. DOI: 10.1378/chest.123.2.387

[43] Enright PL, Sherrill DL. Reference equations for the six minute walk in healthy adults. American Journal of Respiratory and Critical Care Medicine. 1998;**158**:1384-1387. DOI: 10.1164/ajrccm.158.5.9710086

[44] Swigris JJ, Wamboldt FS, Behr J, du Bois RM, King TE, Raghu G, et al. The 6-minute walk in idiopathic pulmonary fibrosis: Longitudinal changes and minimum important difference. Thorax. 2010;**65**:173-177. DOI: 10.1136/thx.2009.113498

[45] Du Bois RM, Weycker D, Albera C, Bradford WZ, Costabel U, Kartashov A, et al. Six minute walk test in idiopathic pulmonary fibrosis. Test validation and minimal clinically important difference. American Journal of Respiratory and Critical Care Medicine. 2011;**183**:1231-1237. DOI: 10.1164/rccm.201007-1179OC

[46] American Thoracic Society, American College of Chest Physicians. ATS/ACCP statement on cardiopulmonary exercise testing. American Journal of Respiratory and Critical Care Medicine. 2003;**167**(2):211-277. DOI: 10.1164/rccm.167.2.211

[47] Gibbons RJ, Balady GJ, Beasley JW, Bricker JT, Duvernoy WF, Froelicher VF, et al. ACC/AHA guidelines for exercise testing: executive summary. A report of the American College of Cardiology. American Heart Association Task Force on Practice Guidelines (Committee on Exercise Testing). Circulation. 1997;**96**:345-354

[48] Bonini M, Fiorenzano G. Exertional dyspnoea in interstitial lung diseases: The clinical utility of cardiopulmonary exercise testing. European Respiratory

Review. 2017;**26**:160099. DOI: 10.1183/16000617.0099-2016

[49] Pitsiou G, Papakosta D, Bouros D. Pulmonary hypertension in idiopathic pulmonary fibrosis: A review. Respiration. 2011;**82**:294-304. DOI: 10.1159/000327918

[50] Manolescu D, Lavinia D, Traila D, Oancea C, Tudorache V. The reliability of lung ultrasound in assessment of idiopathic pulmonary fibrosis. Clinical Interventions in Aging. 2018;**13**:437-449. DOI: 10.2147/CIA.S156615

[51] Lovin S, Veale D. Daily physical activity. In: Tudorache V, Lovin S, Friesen M, editors. Handbook of Pulmonary Rehabilitation. 1st ed. Timisoara: Mirton; 2009. pp. 103-106. ISBN: 978-973-52-0574-4

[52] Nakayama M, Bando M, Araki K, Sekine T, Kurosaki F, Sawata T, et al. Physical activity in patients with idiopathic pulmonary fibrosis. Respirology. 2015;**20**:640-646. DOI: 10.1111/resp.12500

[53] Todea D, Coman A, Rosca L. Tools for assessing the life quality of patients with chronic obstructive pulmonary disease. Clujul Medical. 2012;**85**:20-26

[54] Haskell WL, Lee IM, Pate RR, Powell KE, Blair SN, Franklin BA, et al. Physical activity and public health: Updated recommendation for adults from the American College of Sports Medicine and the American Heart Association. Circulation. 2007;**116**:1081-1093. DOI: 10.1249/mss.0b013e3180616b27

[55] Lee PH, Macfarlane DJ, Lam TH, Stewart SM. Validity of the International Physical Activity Questionnaire Short Form (IPAQ-SF): A systematic review. International Journal of Behavioral Nutrition and Physical Activity. 2011;**8**:115. DOI: 10.1186/1479-5868-8-115

[56] Ryerson CJ, Cayou C, Topp F, Hilling L, Camp PG, Wilcox PG, et al. Pulmonary rehabilitation improves long-term outcomes in interstitial lung disease: a prospective cohort study. Respiratory Medicine. 2014;**108**:203-210. DOI: 10.1016/j.rmed.2013.11.016

[57] Pate RR, Pratt M, Blair SN, Haskell WL, Macera CA, Bouchard C, et al. Physical activity and public health. A recommendation from the Centers for Disease Control and Prevention and the American College of Sports Medicine. JAMA. 1995;**273**:402-407. DOI: 10.1001/jama.1995.03520290054029

[58] Dyrstad SM, Hansen BH, Holme IM, Anderssen SA. Comparison of self-reported versus accelerometer-measured physical activity. Medicine and Science in Sports and Exercise. 2014;**46**(1):99-106. DOI: 10.1249/MSS.0b013e3182a0595f

[59] Mahoney FI, Barthel DW. Functional evaluation: The Barthel index. Maryland State Medical Journal. 1965;**14**:61-65

[60] Lovin S, Veale D. Activities of daily living. In: Tudorache V, Lovin S, Friesen M, editors. Handbook of Pulmonary Rehabilitation. 1st ed. Timisoara: Mirton; 2009. pp. 103-106. ISBN: 978-973-52-0574-4

[61] Pitta F, Troosters T, Probst VS, Spruit MA, Decramer M, Gosselink R. Quantifying physical activity in daily life with questionnaires and motion sensors in COPD. The European Respiratory Journal. 2006;**27**:1040-1055. DOI: 10.1183/09031936.06.00064105

[62] Yorke J, Jones PW, Swigris JJ. Development and validity testing of an IPF-specific version of the St George's Respiratory Questionnaire. Thorax. 2010;**65**(10):921-926. DOI: 10.1136/thx.2010.139121

[63] Jackson RM, Gómez-Marín OW, Ramos CF, Sol CM, Cohen MI, Gaunaurd IA, et al. Exercise limitation in IPF patients: A randomized trial of pulmonary rehabilitation. Lung. 2014;**192**(3):367-376. DOI: 10.1007/s00408-014-9566-9

[64] Grufstedt HK, Shakerand SB, Konradsen H. Validation of the COPD assessment test (CAT) in patients with idiopathic pulmonary fibrosis. European Clinical Respiratory Journal. 2018;**5**:1530028. DOI: 10.1080/20018525.2018.1530028

[65] Ozalevli S, Brazier JE, Harper R, Jones NM, O'Cathain A, Thomas KJ, et al. Validating the SF-36 health survey questionnaire: New outcome measure for primary care. BMJ. 1992;**305**(6846):160-164

[66] Tzanakis N, Maria Samiou T, Lambiri I, Antoniou K, Siafakas N, Bouros D. Evaluation of health related quality of life and dyspnea scales in patients with idiopathic pulmonary fibrosis. Correlation with pulmonary function tests. European Journal of Internal Medicine. 2005;**16**:105-112. DOI: 10.1016/j.ejim.2004.09.013

[67] Chang JA, Randall Curtis J, Patrick DL, Raghu G. Assessment of health-related quality of life in patients with interstitial lung disease. Chest. 1999;**116**(5):1175-1182. DOI: 10.1378/chest.116.5.1175

[68] Sinha A, Patel A, Siegert R, Bajwah S, Keir G, Gordon P, et al. The King's brief interstitial lung disease (K-BILD) questionnaire; an updated minimal important difference. European Respiratory Journal. 2016;**48**:PA808. DOI: 10.1183/13993003.congress-2016.PA808

[69] Dowman L, McDonald CF, Hill CJ, Lee A, Barker K, Boote C, et al. Reliability of the hand held dynamometer in measuring muscle

strength in people with interstitial lung disease. Physiotherapy. 2016;**102**:249-255. DOI: 10.1016/j.physio.2015.10.002

[70] Neder JA, Nery LE, Shinzato GT, Andrade MS, Peres C, Silva AC. Reference values for concentric knee isokinetic strength and power in nonathletic men and women from 20 to 80 years old. The Journal of Orthopaedic and Sports Physical Therapy. 1999;**29**(2):116-126. DOI: 10.2519/jospt.1999.29.2.116

[71] Decramer M, Gosselink R, Troosters T, Verschueren M, Evers G. Muscle weakness is related to utilization of health care resources in COPD patients. The European Respiratory Journal. 1997;**10**(2):417-423. DOI: 10.1183/09031936.97.10020417

[72] Seymour JM, Spruit MA, Hopkinson NS, Natanek SA, Man WD, Jackson A, et al. The prevalence of quadriceps weakness in COPD and the relationship with disease severity. The European Respiratory Journal. 2010;**36**(1):81-88. DOI: 10.1183/09031936.00104909

[73] Nellessen AG, Donária L, Hernandes NA, Pitta F. Analysis of three different equations for predicting quadriceps femoris muscle strength in patients with COPD. Jornal Brasileiro de Pneumologia. 2015;**41**(4):305-312. DOI: 10.1590/S1806-37132015000004515

[74] Caminati A, Bianchi A, Cassandro R, Mirenda MR, Harari S. Walking distance on 6-MWT is a prognostic factor in idiopathic pulmonary fibrosis. Respiratory Medicine. 2009;**103**(1):117-123. DOI: 10.1016/j.rmed.2008.07.022

[75] Tudorache V, Oancea C. Assessments of respiratory muscle strength. In: Tudorache V, Lovin S, Friesen M, editors. Handbook of Pulmonary Rehabilitation. 1st ed. Timisoara: Mirton; 2009. pp. 130-135

[76] Wallaert B, Monge E, Le Rouzic O, Wémeau-Stervinou L, Salleron J, Grosbois JM. Physical activity in daily life of patients with fibrotic idiopathic interstitial pneumonia. Chest. 2013;**144**:1652-1658. DOI: 10.1378/chest.13-0806

[77] Vainshelboim B, Fox BD, Kramer MR, Izhakian S, Gershman E, Oliveira J. Short-term improvement in physical activity and body composition after supervised exercise training program in idiopathic pulmonary fibrosis. Archives of Physical Medicine and Rehabilitation. 2016;**97**(5):788-797. DOI: 10.1016/j.apmr.2016.01.018

[78] Gaunaurd IA, Gomez-Marin OW, Ramos CF, Sol CM, Cohen MI, Cahalin LP, et al. Physical activity and quality of life improvements of patients with idiopathic pulmonary fibrosis completing a pulmonary rehabilitation program. Respiratory Care. 2014;**59**:1872-1879. DOI: 10.4187/respcare.03180

[79] Jastrzebski D, Gumola A, Gawlik R, Kozielski J. Dyspnea and quality of life in patients with pulmonary fibrosis after six weeks of respiratory rehabilitation. Journal of Physiology and Pharmacology. 2006;**57**(Suppl. 4):139-148

[80] Huppmann P, Sczepanski B, Boensch M, Winterkamp S, Schönheit-Kenn U, Neurohr C, et al. Effects of inpatient pulmonary rehabilitation in patients with interstitial lung disease. The European Respiratory Journal. 2013;**42**:444-453. DOI: 10.1183/09031936.00081512

[81] Rammaert B, Leroy S, Cavestri B, Wallaert B, Grosbois JM. Home-based pulmonary rehabilitation in idiopathic pulmonary fibrosis. Revue des Maladies Respiratoires. 2011;**28**:e52-e57. DOI: 10.1016/j.rmr.2011.06.006

[82] Garber CE, Blissmer B, Deschenes MR, Lamonte MJ, Lee IM, Nieman

DC, et al. American College of Sports Medicine position stand. Quantity and quality of exercise for developing and maintaining cardiorespiratory, musculoskeletal, and neuromotor fitness in apparently healthy adults: Guidance for prescribing exercise. Medicine and Science in Sports and Exercise. 2011;**43**:1334-1359. DOI: 10.1249/MSS.0b013e318213fefb

[83] Kozu R, Jenkins S, Senjyu H. Effect of disability level on response to pulmonary rehabilitation in patients with idiopathic pulmonary fibrosis. Respirology. 2011;**16**(8):1196-1202. DOI: 10.1111/j.1440-1843.2011.02029.x

[84] Holland AE, Hill C. Physical training for interstitial lung disease. Cochrane Database of Systematic Reviews. 2008;**4**:10.1002/14651858. CD006322.pub2

[85] Chodzko-Zajko WJ, Proctor DN, Fiatarone Singh MA, Minson CT, Nigg CR, Salem GJ, et al. American College of Sports Medicine position stand. Exercise and physical activity for older adults. Medicine and Science in Sports and Exercise. 2009;**41**:1510-1530. DOI: 10.1249/MSS.0b013e3181a0c95c

[86] Mendoza L, Gogali A, Shrikrishna D, Cavada G, Kemp S, Natanek S, et al. Quadriceps strength and endurance in fibrotic idiopathic interstitial pneumonia. Respirology. 2014;**19**: 138-143. DOI: 10.1111/resp.12181

[87] Mendes P, Wickerson L, Helm D, Janaudis-Ferreira T, Brooks D, Singer L, et al. Skeletal muscle atrophy in advanced interstitial lung disease. Respirology. 2015;**20**:953-959. DOI: 10.1111/resp.12571

[88] American College of Sports Medicine. American College of Sports Medicine position stand. Progression models in resistance training for healthy adults. Medicine and Science in Sports

and Exercise. 2009;**41**:687-708. DOI: 10.1249/MSS.0b013e3181915670

[89] Arizono S, Taniguchi H, Sakamoto K, Kondoh Y, Kimura T, Kataoka K, et al. Endurance time is the most responsive exercise measurement in idiopathic pulmonary fibrosis. Respiratory Care. 2014;**59**:1108-1115. DOI: 10.4187/respcare.02674

[90] Markovitz GH, Cooper CB. Mechanisms of exercise limitation and pulmonary rehabilitation for patients with pulmonary fibrosis/restrictive lung disease. Chronic Respiratory Disease. 2010;**7**(1):47-60. DOI: 10.1177/1479972309348654

[91] Cyrino ES, Okano AH, Glaner MF, Romanzini M, Gobbo LA, Makoski A, et al. Impact of the use of different skinfold calipers for the analysis of the body composition. Revista Brasileira de Medicina do Esporte. 2003;**9**:150-153. DOI: 10.1590/S1517-86922003000300004

[92] Pollock M, Gaesser GA, Butcher JD, Després JP, Dishman RK, Franklin BA, et al. American College of Sports Medicine Position Stand. The recommended quantity and quality of exercise for developing and maintaining cardiorespiratory and muscular fitness, and flexibility in healthy adults. Medicine & Science in Sports & Exercise. 1998;**30**:975-991

[93] Chéhère B, Bougault V, Chenivesse C, Grosbois JM, Wallaert B. Cardiorespiratory adaptation in a 6-minute walk test by fibrotic idiopathic interstitial pneumonia patients who did or did not respond to pulmonary rehabilitation. European Journal of Physical and Rehabilitation Medicine. 2018. DOI: 10.23736/S1973-9087.18.05093-1

[94] https://www.ishlt.org/ The International Society for Heart & Lung Transplantation

[95] Wickerson L, Rozenberg D, Janaudis-Ferreira T, Deliva R, Lo V, Beauchamp G, et al. Physical rehabilitation for lung transplant candidates and recipients: An evidence-informed clinical approach. World Journal of Transplantation. 2016;**6**(3):517-531. DOI: 10.5500/wjt. v6.i3.517

[96] Weill D, Benden C, Corris PA, Dark JH, Davis RD, Keshavjee S, et al. A consensus document for the selection of lung transplant candidates: 2014—An update from the Pulmonary Transplantation Council of the International Society for Heart and Lung Transplantation. The Journal of Heart and Lung Transplantation. 2015;**34**(1):1-15. DOI: 10.1016/j. healun.2014.06.014

www.ingramcontent.com/pod-product-compliance
Lightning Source LLC
Chambersburg PA
CBHW081238190326
41458CB00016B/5833